T0356027

THE PROTEIN PLAYBOOK

Build Strength, Boost Metabolism & Feel Energized

HEARST
HOME

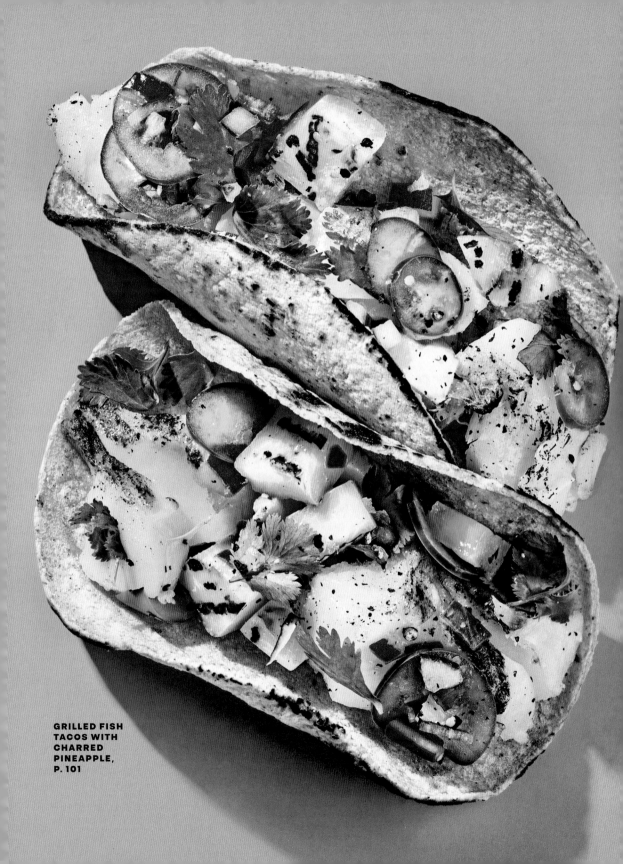

GRILLED FISH TACOS WITH CHARRED PINEAPPLE, P. 101

Contents

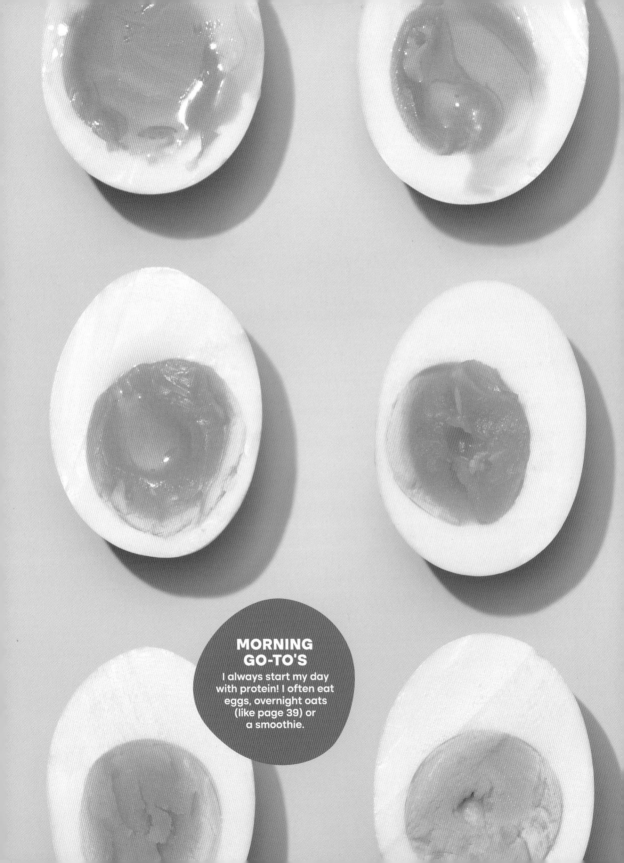

MORNING GO-TO'S

I always start my day with protein! I often eat eggs, overnight oats (like page 39) or a smoothie.

The Power of Protein

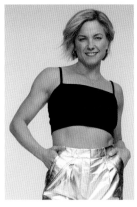

I've been writing and editing nutrition, health, and fitness articles for more than 20 years. So I've known for a long time how crucial protein is to our health and well-being, particularly for women.

And yet! Some hardwired habits from childhood kept me stuck in my low-fat, avoid-meat ways until a couple years ago. I decided to see how much protein I was consuming on an average day. It wasn't much...around 50g, or half the amount many experts recommend for an active woman like me who works out five days a week.

From there, I began to truly prioritize protein. That meant reading nutrition levels, using a food scale, and for a while, logging my daily protein consumption in a food tracker app and aiming for at least 30g of protein in every meal. Eventually, I was eating 100 to 125g every day. Everything felt better: more energy, faster recovery from workouts, sounder sleep.

Now I can look at a chicken breast and mentally calculate how much protein it contains. I don't count calories or other macros because I find that, for me, when I prioritize protein, everything else falls into place. The I-feel-soooo-good effects were delightful, but I'll admit that the aesthetic changes I noticed in my body were also motivating (hello, abs!).

Since then, I haven't stopped singing the benefits from the rooftops to anyone who will listen, including *Women's Health* readers. I want every woman to experience the powerful impact protein makes in how you feel, how you show up in your life...and how good you feel as you age.

I have a big job and three kiddos plus a dog and a husband, so you better believe that everything in the pages that follow is meant to help you fit protein—hacks, recipes, meal-prep tips, protein powder suggestions, and so much more—into your already very-busy life.

LIZ BAKER PLOSSER
EDITOR-IN-CHIEF
@ @lizplosser

PART ONE

Why Protein Matters

Protein is a key macronutrient that claims **superhero status** but, until very recently, tended not to be a priority until dinner. But experts say that when you start focusing on eating more protein at every meal (and snack) throughout the day, good things tend to follow.

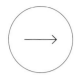

Protein is so freakin' awesome because... "Besides muscle strength, performance, and aesthetics, protein plays a huge role in our overall metabolic balance," says *Women's Health* advisor Lauren Kanski, CPT, kettlebell expert and senior founding fitness and nutrition coach for the Ladder app. "It is also the most satiating macro, and consuming adequate protein and improving muscle health decreases blood pressure, lowers blood sugar, decreases triglycerides, increases HDL, strengthens immune function, the list goes on..."

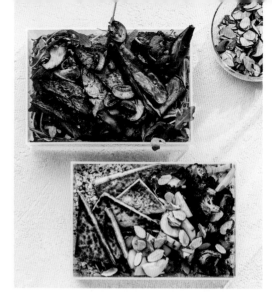

Still, it isn't quite as easy as just eating more steak (sorry!), especially if you want to ensure a balanced, nutrient-dense diet. The best protein sources—fish, lean meats, dairy, beans—may not seem as quick and easy to add to your day as carbs, fruits, and veggies. That may help explain why up to a third of women between the ages of 20 and 40 don't get their recommended daily amount of protein, according to data from the U.S. Department of Agriculture. Plus, a growing number of nutritionists believe that the current dietary guidelines for this mighty macronutrient are way too low, and we're really missing out.

Consider this: A Johns Hopkins University study found that a diet in which roughly a quarter of the calories (about 60 percent more than the recommended 10 to 15 percent) come from lean protein sources reduced blood pressure, LDL ("bad") cholesterol levels, and triglycerides better than a traditional higher-carb diet. Other research finds that diets rich in protein can help prevent obesity, osteoporosis, and diabetes.

Okay, so clearly there's something to eating a diet that's packed with protein. For now, here's what you need to know about eating a high-protein diet and how to make it work for you.

Protein and Your Body

Many high-protein foods are often more calorie-dense than many high-carb foods, like fruits and veggies, so it might seem a little counterintuitive that a high-protein diet can help with weight management.

But here's the thing: High-protein foods take more work to digest, metabolize, and convert to energy in your body, which means you burn more calories processing them. They also take longer to digest so they keep you feeling full for a longer amount of time. The cumulative effect has obvious benefits for anyone who is watching their weight. In a study published in the *Journal of Nutrition and Metabolism*, dieters who increased their protein intake to 30 percent of their diet ate nearly 450 fewer calories a day and lost about 11 pounds over the 12-week study without employing any other dietary measures.

Your body also uses the amino acids in protein to build lean muscle, which not only makes you stronger but also burns calories even when you're not active. Ultimately, this keeps your metabolism humming along at high speed all day long.

But there's more to protein than just metabolism and muscle: "People tend to only think of muscle and protein in relation to fitness, and that's a mistake," says Gabrielle Lyon, DO, founder of Muscle-Centric Medicine. When you eat protein, the amino acids that are present are the "building blocks of life," explains Cara Harbstreet, MS, RD, LD, a registered dietitian and owner of Street Smart Nutrition.

Humans need amino acids to perform essential functions throughout the body. This means they help mount a response to infection, as well as for just about every structure in the body—

bone, liver, gut, tissues, hair, nails, skin—and act as enzymes, hormones, buffers, transporters, and regulators, she says.

Skin and aging are also intertwined with protein. "Every organ, from the lungs to the liver to our largest, the skin, is made up of thousands of different proteins," says Michael Sherratt, PhD, a professor of biochemistry at the University of Manchester in England. Some are unique to their location; others, like collagen, can be found in multiple areas, like your bones, connective tissue, and, of course, your skin. Then there are specialized proteins like fibrillin (which helps keep skin bouncy), fibronectin (essential to tissue repair), and laminin (involved in healing damage). Experts advise an inside-out approach—read: eating a varied diet rich in proteins—to ensure you have the proteins you need to keep skin strong.

Over the past 20 years, researchers have come to understand that skeletal muscles are endocrine organs, just like the thyroid. During muscle contraction, they produce and secrete small proteins, called myokines, that can keep inflammation from getting out of hand. This is also why being under-muscled is fast becoming a health problem to watch.

But this whole convo isn't about how much you can deadlift; patients with less muscle mass have more complications, longer hospital stays, and lower survival rates, according to an *Annals of Medicine* review of nearly 150 studies. Plus, aging bodies process protein less efficiently and need more of it to maintain muscle strength, bone health, and other functions.

Start thinking of muscle as a healthy aging strategy, beyond the aesthetic aspect, suggests Dr. Lyon. One way to do that: Focus on high-quality protein, she says, which will protect you from many chronic diseases.

"Humans can synthesize, or create, some of the amino acids needed to build complex proteins. However, we must source essential amino acids that we can't make ourselves from our diets," Harbstreet says. "Eating a variety of foods, both plant- and animal-based, can ensure you eat enough total protein as well as sources for all essential amino acids."

What the Pros Know

Athletes and team dietitians share their most valuable high-protein meals.

"My favorite high-protein meal... is taking Greek yogurt, adding a little dollop of honey and cut peaches and watermelon. Maybe some blueberries and granola on top. Peaches and watermelon you wouldn't normally think to put on top of Greek yogurt, but it is so refreshing and delicious."
—*Scout Bassett, paralympic track athlete*

"I love making bowls with chicken and chickpeas, because chickpeas are great sources of protein, and you get it from the chicken too. And then you can add some rice in there. So it's a protein-packed meal, super easy."
—*Katie Ahlers, team dietitian for the Los Angeles Rams*

"I'm a simple girl. Fish, I would say. Some nice grilled salmon."
–*Allyson Felix, most decorated female track and field athlete*

"Definitely salmon and mashed potatoes."
—*Aliyah Boston, WNBA power forward for the Indiana Fever and 2023 Rookie of the Year*

How Much Protein Do I Need?

Listen up: Experts are (loudly) singing protein's praises.
If you have ever wondered, "am I getting enough?" or questioned
what the best protein sources are, here's the answer.

While the recommended daily allowance, a.k.a. the RDA, from the Food and Nutrition Board of the National Academy of Sciences has long held at 0.8 grams per kilogram of body weight (or 0.36 grams per pound), other experts stress that women and those who are active likely need *much* more than that.

"That is just a baseline," says Kristen Smith, RD, a national spokesperson for the Academy of Nutrition and Dietetics. "It's the minimum amount you need to eat daily to stay healthy but doesn't take into account specific goals or medical conditions," she says.

Many researchers are now saying we need more like 1.2 to 1.5 grams per kilogram to support tissue growth. (Especially if you exercise regularly!) In practice, for example, a 140-pound person should be eating at least 76 to 95 grams total per day.

But most of us don't have the time or the energy to meticulously calculate our macros for every meal of the day. An easier way to hit your target? Aim for about 20 to 30 grams per meal. And FYI: the "per meal" language is intentional; you really do need to eat it all day.

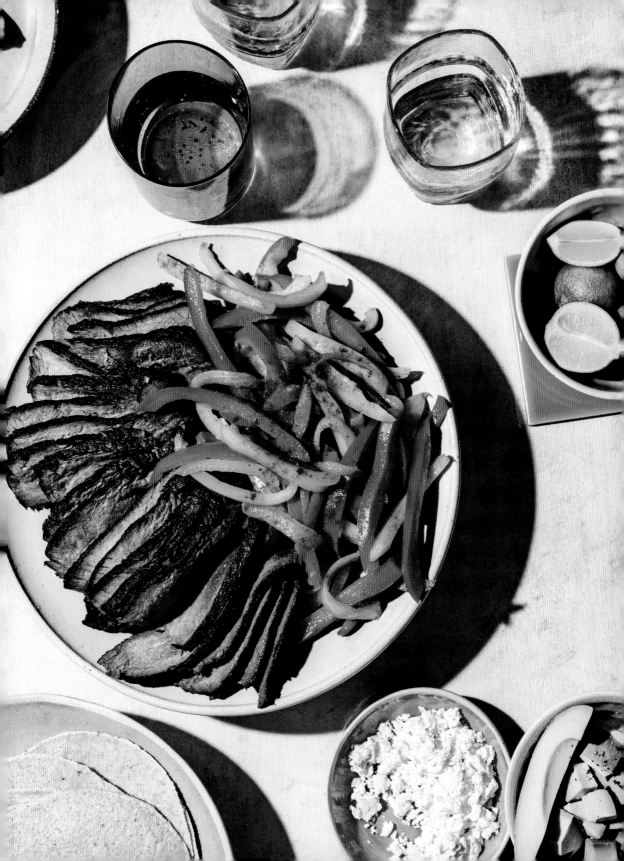

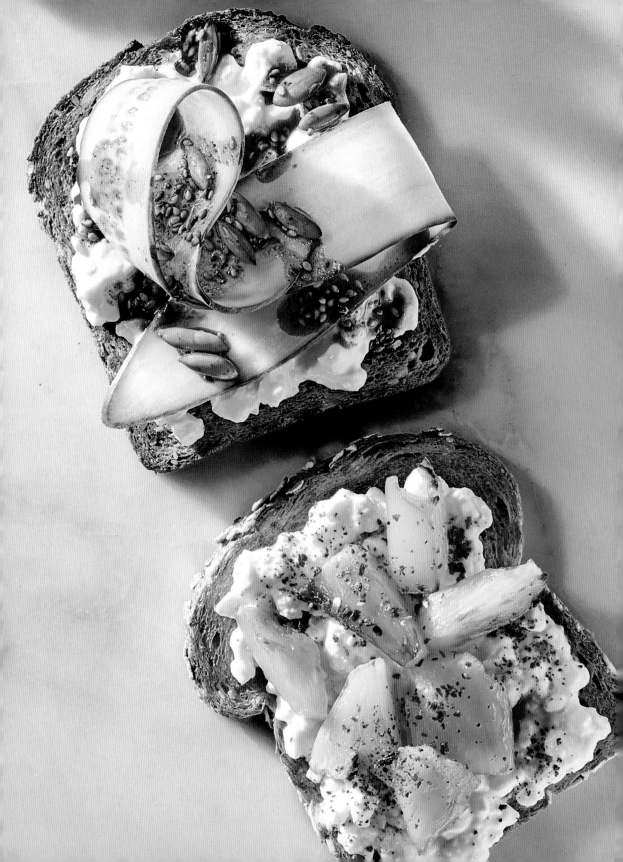

That's because the body doesn't store amino acids. While extra carbohydrates are stored in the body as glycogen and surplus fat is stored as body fat, amino acids aren't squirreled away to be used later. Rather, after our body uses what it can of the protein we eat at a meal—to support metabolism, produce hormones, maintain bones and, yes, aid muscle protein synthesis—it is then converted into either fat or glucose. That means it's best to have protein available at any time, so spread your proteins throughout the day—including breakfast, of course.

The Best Time for Protein (Hint: All the Time)

Generally speaking, the time of day during which you consume protein doesn't matter, in and of itself, as much as how you distribute your intake throughout the day.

If you're like most Americans, you're probably getting the bulk of your protein at dinner. Women between the ages of 20 and 49 were found, on average, to consume about 42 percent of their daily protein at dinner and just 17 percent at breakfast, per a survey conducted by the U.S. Department of Agriculture's (USDA) Agriculture Research Service.

What we should be aiming for instead is an equal distribution of protein throughout the day, say experts. Research shows spreading out protein intake every three to four hours or so into moderate doses versus eating it all at once is associated with more optimal muscle repair—and for those who are looking for growth, more optimal growth too.

Moreover, research seems to indicate that around 20 to 30 grams of protein at one time is the amount that our body can use for muscle synthesis. Essentially, anything over that in a single meal may not make a huge difference as far as protein actions in the body go.

Another reason you may want to consider spacing out your protein throughout the day instead of cramming it all in at dinner? You'll probably get less hungry throughout the day.

Your Ideal Day in Protein

See what a "perfect" day of protein might look like and do your best to meet these goals whenever you can.

morning

● Planning on waking up and getting in an early workout? Nibble on a banana beforehand to stabilize your blood sugar.
● Post-workout (or your first food of the day if you didn't exercise), try a veggie omelet and a slice of avocado toast.
● Three hours later, if it isn't time for lunch, have a snack of peanuts or pistachios with a side of crackers and hummus, or pair the nuts with a small piece of fruit.

afternoon

● Cook up either a chicken breast or a salmon filet (or, if you prefer a plant-based protein, tofu), and a side of cooked vegetables and quinoa. Another alternative: Throw the protein and quinoa on top of a bed of lettuce for a salad and add a little dressing.
● If you're someone who eats a later dinner, you'll once again want a snack in between meals; go for roasted edamame with some raisins.

evening

● For your final meal of the day, opt for a protein you haven't had yet (either one of the above or shrimp) paired with farro (a higher-protein grain) and some roasted broccoli (also a a high-protein veggie!).

Of course, these are just suggestions and everybody's body will respond to protein amounts and timings differently. Before settling on a plan, experiment to find out what works best for you and your specific goals. "You can try playing with timing; you can try dosing a little higher and a little lower within that range and see how you feel," says Tracy Anthony, PhD, a professor of nutritional science at Rutgers University in New Brunswick, New Jersey.

People notice that when they start to emphasize protein at breakfast and they ensure that it's there at their snack too, they feel more satiated throughout the day and are less likely to have blood sugar spikes and crashes.

Understanding Complete and Incomplete Protein

Okay, let's take a beat to jump back into some basic science here. Protein in general is made up of lots of amino acids. Amino acids are the building blocks for growing and repairing our body's tissues, as well as many other important functions that keep our body working properly.

Some amino acids are considered "nonessential," meaning our body can produce them on its own if we don't get enough through the protein-rich foods that we eat. But there are other amino acids that we can't naturally produce—nine of them, to be exact. Complete proteins contain all nine of those essential amino acids that we must get through food.

Like you've probably guessed by now, incomplete proteins don't contain those nine essential amino acids. These types of proteins are still important to consume, though, because they often have complementary amino acids that your body needs.

Which is better? Neither! You need both types to keep your muscles strong and support good collagen production. You don't need to worry about eating certain essential amino acids at every meal. Instead, focus on getting a balance of protein sources over the course of the day.

Post-Workout Protein Is Especially Important

It's key to eat protein after a sweat sesh. Perhaps you've heard the term anabolic or metabolic window? This refers to the time period after exercise in which your muscles are repairing themselves and nutrition can play a role in aiding that process

Thankfully, research shows that the window is about three or four hours after a workout. As for the amount of protein, aim for 20 to 25 grams post-workout, recommends Tracy Anthony, PhD, a professor of nutritional sciences at Rutgers University in New Brunswick, New Jersey.

Also important to note: If all of this talk about post-workout fueling has you wondering about pre-workout fueling, we have that answer too. If you're exercising for an hour or less, you probably don't need to worry about protein intake ahead of time and can simply focus on getting high-quality protein after. However, if you're going for, say, a two-hour run or you tend to feel peckish if you don't eat before exercising, grab a carb-rich snack with a few grams of protein first. "It will help a little bit with your energy levels and reduce the amount of muscle damage you're going to have go on there too," Jones says.

MORE PROTEIN TIPS

■ If you're vegan, vegetarian, or pescatarian, prioritize complete plant-based proteins like quinoa and soy.

■ If eggs, fish, and cheese fit into your eating style, those are smart complete proteins to build into your meals as well.

■ Try rice and beans or whole wheat bread with peanut butter for a meal or snack that's full of complementary proteins.

■ Don't forget protein powders. Flip to page 24 for more.

Types of Proteins

Besides complete and incomplete, proteins also fall into two main categories: animal proteins and plant proteins. Below is a cheat sheet of *Women's Health* editors' favorite protein sources (including serving size and macros) within these categories.

ANIMAL PROTEIN provides all nine of the essential amino acids and is great as part of your main course.

- **Eggs** 1 egg: 6 grams protein
- **Cottage cheese** ¹/₂ cup: 14 grams protein
- **Greek yogurt** 6 ounces: 18 grams protein
- **Chicken breast** 4 ounces: 33 grams protein
- **Beef jerky** 1 cup: 30 grams protein
- **Ground turkey** 1 cup: 30 grams protein
- **Salmon** 5 ounces: 35 grams protein

PLANT PROTEIN is rich in fiber but it's slightly less digestible and contains fewer essential amino acids than animal protein. As a result, plant protein requires some mixing and matching to reach the necessary amino acids your body needs, so you'll need to eat more of it to cover your bases.

- **Edamame** 1 cup: 31 grams protein
- **Lentils** 1 cup: 22 grams protein
- **Black beans** 2 cups: 30 grams protein
- **Nuts and seeds** 1 ounce: 4 to 9 grams protein
- **Peas** 1 cup: 8 grams protein
- **Quinoa** ¹/₂ cup: 4 grams protein
- **Chickpeas** ¹/₂ cup: 7 grams protein
- **Tofu** 3 ounces: 9 grams protein

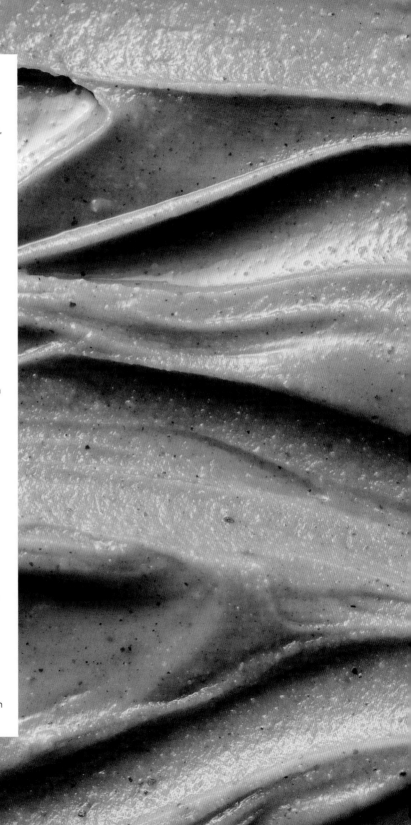

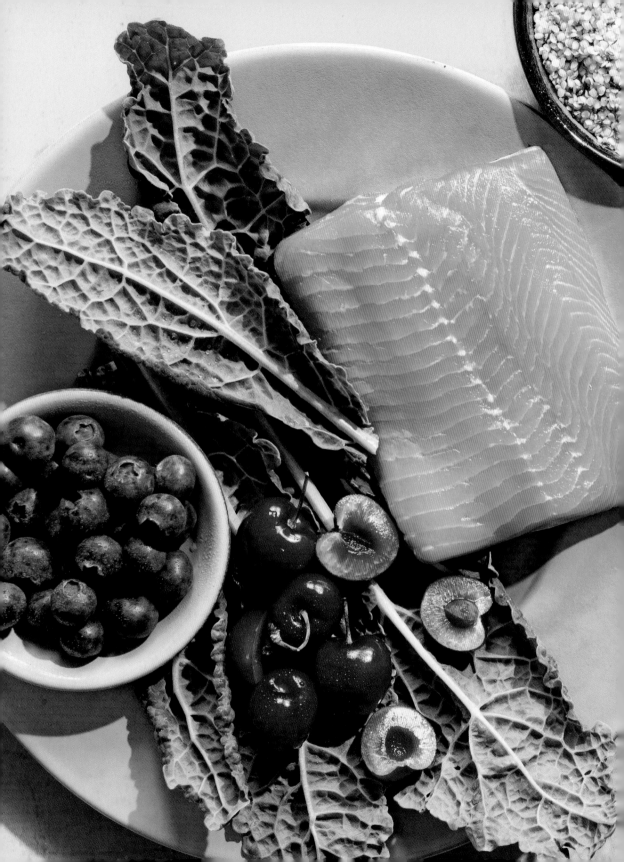

The Best Sources

How to pick protein throughout every single grocery aisle.

So you've decided to prioritize protein in your diet. Congrats! You're one step closer to building muscle and boosting satiety all day long. You already know you need to eat foods that contain protein, because while the body synthesizes many amino acids that make up protein chains, there are some the body can't make up.

After that, there's a lot of back and forth about how much your body needs, in what form (animal, vegetable, or vanilla-flavored white powder poured in a giant plastic container to be sold at the supplement shop), and whether the macronutrient itself can help you lose weight or build more muscle.

When it comes to the protein publicity machine, chicken, beef, and pork tend to hog (no pun intended!) the limelight. And it's easy to see why: Not only do animal products provide all nine essential amino acids, but their protein counts, gram for gram, are hard to beat (one T-bone steak boasts a jaw-dropping 98 grams of protein!). It's no wonder that steers walk around with all that main-character energy.

Jokes aside, the longtime supporting player, plant-based protein, is also a great source of protein. In fact, it's really starting to come into its own. Industry experts project that the plant-based protein market could account for nearly 8 percent of the global protein market by 2030 (from a value of nearly $30 billion in 2020 up to $162 billion), thanks to the growing number of options and the ease with which consumers can find plant-based products at stores and restaurants. And even if you're not vegan or vegetarian, there are a number of reasons to embrace plant-based protein as part of your diet (for more, turn to page 22).

The good news is that these days, you can find this essential nutrient in ingredients and products in nearly every section of the grocery store. Let us give you a tour of some of the protein-rich (and delicious) choices available.

The Dairy Aisle
Cottage cheese, yogurt, cheese, eggs, and milk: all protein star players. Consider skyr, a creamy Icelandic yogurt made from strained cheese (similar to Greek yogurt, but thicker and less tangy), which has 21 grams of protein per serving.

The Bakery Department
Carbs don't leap to mind when you're looking for protein-packed foods. But keep an eye out for fortified breads, wraps, and crackers with added protein that can help bulk up a sandwich or salad. Some have up to 15 grams of protein and 5 grams of dietary fiber.

The Produce Section
Fresh vegetables aren't always super high in protein, but there are some that contain more than others. Avocados, for example, aren't prized only for their creamy texture and toast compatibility—a medium-size one also has about 3 grams of protein. And don't sleep on a great meat substitute, mushrooms—though not all are created equal. Shitake mushrooms have 2.3 grams in one cup, versus 3 grams in basic white button. Keep an eye out for tofu and soy protein options—typically shelved with produce. For more high-protein veggies, turn to page 149.

Cereal and Dry Goods
Look for breakfast-cereal options that feature added plant-based protein. For instance, some brands contain pea protein—specifically the protein in yellow split peas. Plus, don't forget about oatmeal! This is also where you're going to come across nuts, a great source of protein. (That's one of the reasons so many granola and protein bars use nuts and nut butters as a base— and you can pick up these here as well.) But don't

48%
The number of consumers who said they knew how much protein they'd had in the past 24 hours.

Source: FMCG. Gurus survey.

glide by the tinned fish, beef jerky, and boxed broths. Stock up on lentils, quinoa, beans, and other high-protein pantry staples.

The Meat/Fish Counter
This one may feel like a no-brainer, since red meat is obviously high in protein, but try shaking up your routine with something different. Take advantage of your butcher's knowledge, and diversify your meat consumption beyond beef, chicken, and pork with lamb, turkey, and lean game meats. On the fish front, consider trout, salmon, and mackerel, as well as mussels, oysters and shrimp, for well-rounded, healthy options.

Frozen Foods
This aisle is a gold mine for protein-packed items that can last for months in the freezer and be tossed into any dish—from chicken nuggets to faux chicken nuggets, as well as soy, tempeh, and other plant-based proteins that come in as many forms as you can imagine (burgers, grounds, links).

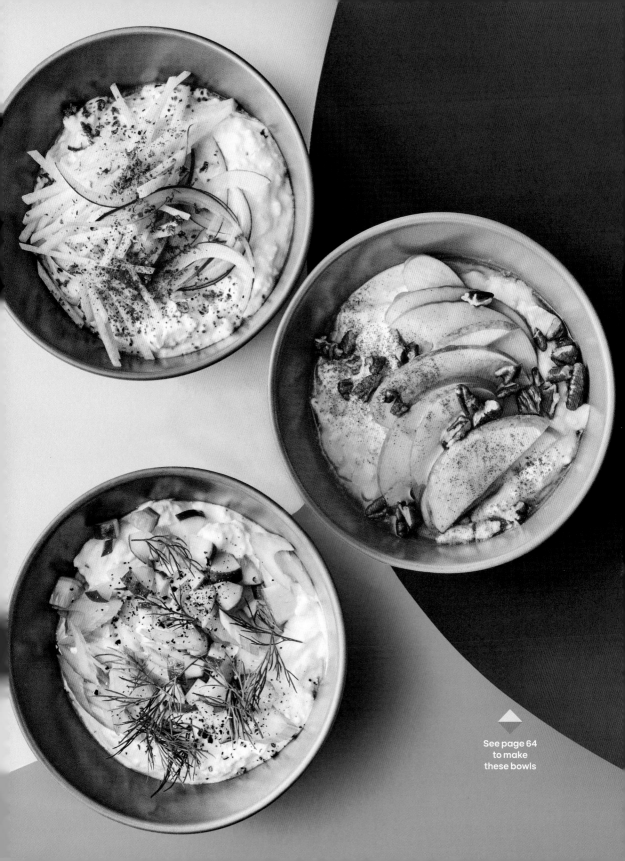

See page 64
to make
these bowls

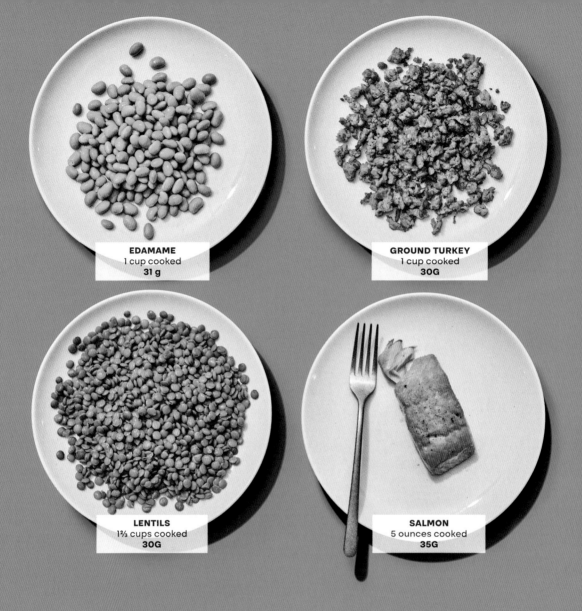

EDAMAME
1 cup cooked
31 g

GROUND TURKEY
1 cup cooked
30G

LENTILS
1⅓ cups cooked
30G

SALMON
5 ounces cooked
35G

What Does 30g of Protein Look Like?

If you're trying to increase your protein intake or simply eat more protein at every meal, looking for high-protein foods that give you a lot of protein bang for your buck is one smart strategy that can help. However, it's good to know what volume of said food you need to consume to hit a number like 20 to 30 grams per meal. Here's what it looks like on a plate.

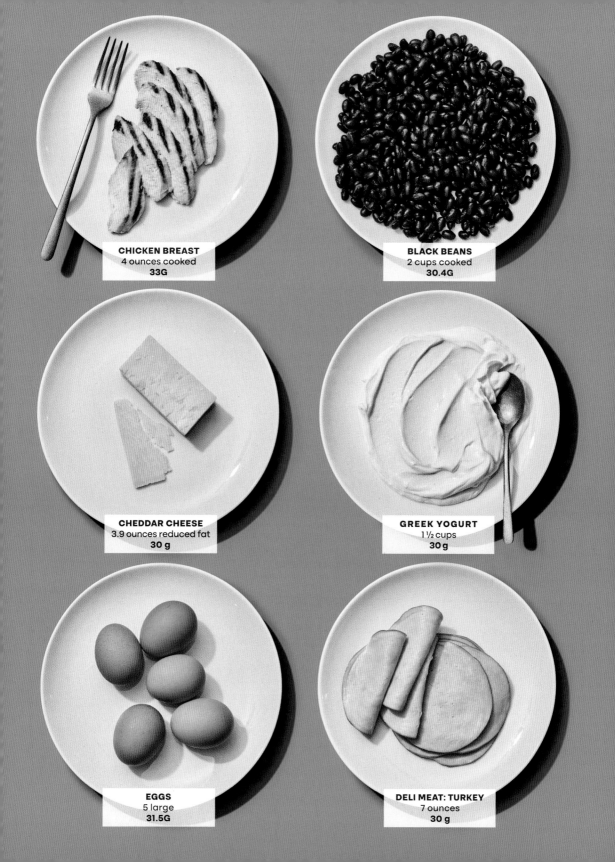

CHICKEN BREAST
4 ounces cooked
33G

BLACK BEANS
2 cups cooked
30.4G

CHEDDAR CHEESE
3.9 ounces reduced fat
30 g

GREEK YOGURT
1 ½ cups
30 g

EGGS
5 large
31.5G

DELI MEAT: TURKEY
7 ounces
30 g

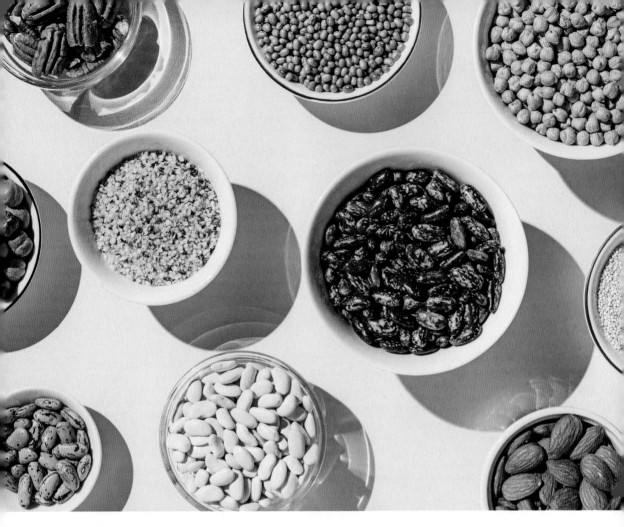

Plant Power

A well-rounded diet includes many varieties of plant-based foods, including grains, legumes, and seeds. These are the best sources to meet your protein goals.

BLACK BEANS

Beans may not be the best option if you're following a high-protein, low-carb diet, but if you're looking for a base for some vegetarian chili or tacos, black beans are hard to beat. Plus, studies have shown that they may also help lower cholesterol.

Per serving (1 cup, boiled with salt) *227 calories, 0.93 g fat (0.24 g saturated), 40.8 g carbs, 0.55 g sugar, 408 mg sodium, 15 g fiber, 15.2 g protein*

CHIA SEEDS

These first became popular with the much-hyped chia seed pudding, but there are plenty of other ways to add this superfood into your diet. Mix them into your favorite homemade treats, create chia tea, or whip them with water for an egg alternative when baking.

Per serving (1 oz) *138 calories, 8.7 g fat (0.94 g saturated), 11.9 g carbs, 0 g sugar, 4.54 mg sodium, 9.75 g fiber, 4.68 g protein*

CHICKPEAS

From starring in Mediterranean dishes like hummus to adding a great source of protein to curries to sneaking their way into vegan brownies, is there anything chickpeas can't do? Not only are they filled with protein, but chickpeas are also a great source of fiber.

Per serving (1 cup) *269 calories, 4.25 g fat (0.44 g saturated), 44.9 g carbs, 7.87 g sugar, 11.5 mg sodium, 12.5 g fiber, 14.5 g protein*

FLAXSEED

You can buy flax whole or ground, and both are super handy choices. Flaxseed is a great source of heart-healthy omega-3s, which can help protect against chronic diseases like cancer and heart disease. Stir whole flaxseed into oatmeal for crunch or use ground flaxseed in baked goods like cookies and pie crusts.

Per serving (1 oz) *150 calories, 12 g fat (1 g saturated), 8 mg sodium, 8 g carbs, 0.5 G fiber, 7.5 G sugar, 5 g protein*

HEMP SEEDS

Mixing in or sprinkling a tablespoon or two of hemp hearts into your meals will give you an extra boost of protein, fiber, and magnesium.

Per serving (3 tbsp) *166 calories, 14.6 g fat (1.38 g saturated), 2.6 g carbs, 0.45 g sugar, 1.5 mg sodium, 1.2 g fiber, 9.48 g protein, 8 g protein*

KIDNEY BEANS

These tasty little guys have many benefits, including reducing cholesterol and lowering blood-sugar levels.

Per serving (1 cup) *222 calories, 0 g fat (0 g saturated), 42 g carbs, 619 mg sodium, 6 g sugar, 16 g fiber, 14 g protein*

LENTILS

You probably recognize these little legumes from the bulk section at your grocery store, and that's also where you're likely to get them for the best deal. Next time you're making soup or hankering for a good homemade veggie burger, lentils—whether you go with brown, green, or red—are a good place to start.

Per serving (1 cup) *230 calories, 8 g fat (.1 G saturated), 40 g carbs, 3.6 g sugar, 4 mg sodium, 16 g fiber, 18 g protein*

NUTRITIONAL YEAST

Any underrated powerhouse, nutritional yeast contains all nine essential amino acids, B vitamins, and antioxidants.

Per serving (¼ cup): *60 calories, 0.5 g fat (0 g saturated), 5 g carbs, 25 mg sodium, 0 g sugar, 3 g fiber, 8 g protein*

OATS

If eggs are a no-go in the a.m. for you, overnight oats are your BFF. They are a good choice for your morning meal because, in addition to their protein content, they contain fiber—specifically beta-glucan, which has been shown to lower cholesterol.

Per serving (1 cup) *150 calories, 2.5 g fat (0.5 g saturated), 27 g carbs, 0 mg sodium, 1 g sugar, 4 g fiber, 5 g protein*

SEITAN

Made from wheat protein, seitan has a savory, nutty taste (but it will absorb the flavors of whatever it's cooked with) and a stringy texture that's almost, dare you say it, meat-like.

Per serving (2.5 oz) *90 calories, 1 g fat (0 g saturated), 4 g carbs, 2 g sugar, 340 mg sodium, 1 g fiber, 17 g protein*

TEMPEH

If you're all about those complete plant proteins, tempeh is a must. This fermented soy food is packed with flavor and may lend a probiotic boost. Try marinating sliced tempeh in grated ginger and soy sauce and then searing it in a wok with peppers, onions, and broccoli for a satisfying stir-fry.

Per serving (6 slices) *140 calories, 3.5 g fat (0 g saturated), 40 g carbs, 4 mg sodium, 4 g sugar, 16 g fiber, 11 g protein*

TOFU

There's a good reason why you'll see a number of soy-based options on this list. The bean itself offers all of the essential amino acids your body craves, packing a protein punch akin to that in animal-based foods. Tofu, a bean curd made from soy, has been a popular protein-rich alternative for decades. Taking the time to marinate it or season it will help make it the star of any dish.

Per serving (100 g) *76 calories, 4.8 g fat (.7 g saturated), 1.9 g carbs, 0 g sugar, 7 mg sodium, .3 g fiber, 8 g protein*

QUINOA

An ancient grain packed with nutrients, quinoa also offers all nine essential amino acids your body needs. Use it as a base for your fave bowl at lunch (and save yourself dropping $20 at that fancy salad place) or sub it in when recipes call for other grains.

Per serving (1 cup cooked) *222 calories, 3.55 g fat (0.43 G saturated), 39.4 g carbs, 1.61 g sugar, 13 mg sodium, 5.18 g fiber, 8.14 g protein*

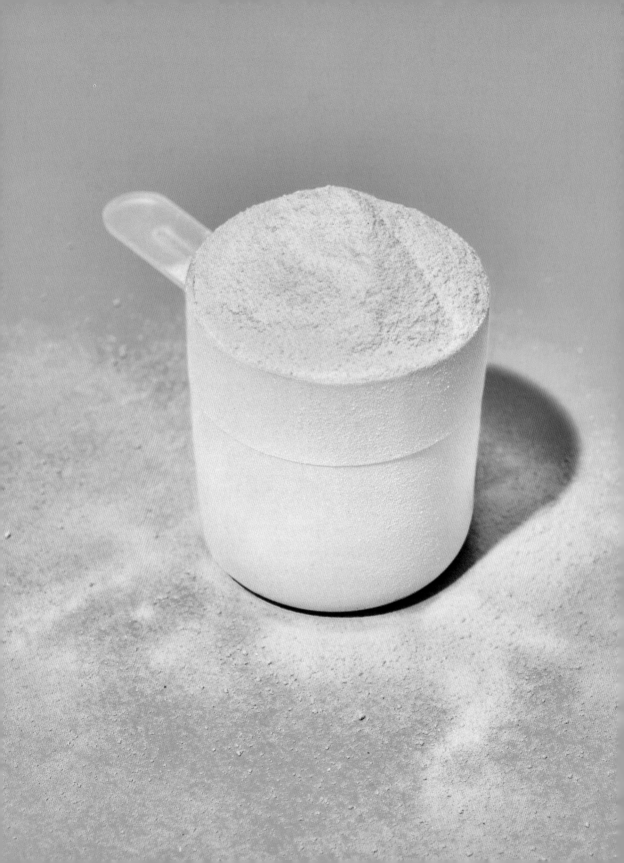

All About Protein Powders

Meeting protein goals with food alone can be tough for some people. This supplement offers a little extra help.

→

While most trainers and dietitians will recommend whole foods first to hit your nutrient needs, there's not always time to whip up a real meal. Enter protein powder. "It's a very convenient way to get a decent amount of protein in a small amount of time," says Dana White, RD, a registered dietitian and athletic trainer who specializes in sports nutrition.

That's just the beginning. "When you eat is really just as important as what you eat," says White. That's especially true for protein. Unlike other macronutrients (carbs and fat), you're not able to store protein. That means your body needs a consistent stream of it coming in. (One protein-packed meal a day will not cut it.)

What is protein powder?

There is no one-size-fits-all protein powder definition, but "'isolated protein supplement' is probably the best way to describe it," says White. The powder you scoop out of the tub is extracted from a protein-rich food and converted into the mixable form. There are a variety of different animal- and plant-based protein powders.

While animal-based protein powders will likely be a single source (like whey, casein, or collagen), plant-based protein powders are generally a blend of different plant proteins (soy, hemp, pea, rice, and more). "Out of the 20 amino acids that exist, there are nine essential amino acids that you can only get from food," says White. "Animal-based foods have all nine essential amino acids, whereas plant-based proteins are lacking one or more of those nine essential amino acids." (FYI: Soy is the only plant-based protein that includes all essential amino acids; the rest need to be combined to deliver the essential amino acids.)

When you think of protein powder, you probably conjure images of colorful shaker bottles and gym bros. And if so, you'd be vastly underestimating the power of the powder and the ways you can use it. Flip the page for a few top tips and delicious recipes that use protein powder.

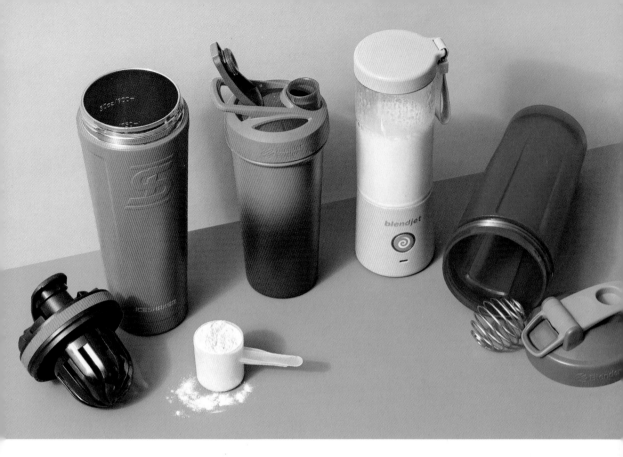

Whip Up Protein Pancakes
You can buy already-mixed protein pancake mix, or you can DIY them by adding a scoop of powder to your fave recipe. Try our recipe on page 37!

Optimize Gluten-Free Baking
If you're baking with gluten-free flours, whey protein powder helps to provide some of the structure and texture to the flour that gluten would normally provide. If you switch to almond flour from all-purpose flour, you could have a crumbly mess unless you use something—like whey—that's going to mimic gluten.

Make Overnight Oats
Divide 1 single-serve Greek yogurt between two mason jars. Then add to each jar: 1 scoop protein powder, ¼ cup raw oats, and ¾ cups liquid.

Sip the Perfect Recovery Shake
If you mix protein powder with water post-workout, it probably won't have enough carbohydrate to support good muscle growth. To add the necessary carbs (and replenish your body's glycogen stores used up in your sweat sesh), mix 1 scoop powder with milk or juice, or grab a banana on the side. Looking for something a bit more substantial? Try a Super Shake: Super shakes are essentially a meal in a glass that includes high-quality liquid nutrition that gives you everything you need in a convenient, portable, delicious package. Basically, you choose a liquid, protein powder, veggie, fruit, healthy fat, and a "topper" (i.e. cocoa nibs or coconut), then blend and enjoy.

Try It Anytime, Anywhere
An unflavored protein power is perfect to mix into almost any type of food to boost your macro count. Sprinkle some into pasta sauce, soups, salad dressing, yogurt, dips, and more.

Our Protein Powder Picks

It may take a bit of trial and error to find a protein powder that you like, and it can feel like there are a million powders on the market. Here are the ones that our editors and testers liked the best, in various categories.

BEST FOR BAKING
ALOHA Organic Plant-Based Protein Powder
It contains a blend of organic pea, organic brown rice, organic pumpkin seed, and organic hemp seed protein to hit all the essential amino acids. Monk fruit extract provides just enough sweetness without artificial sweeteners or excess sugar. It's versatile and works well blended in a smoothie or added to baked goods, like muffins and cookies, to up the protein content.

BEST VEGETARIAN
Orgain Organic Vegan Protein Powder
Pea, brown rice, and chia seed form the base for this plant-based protein powder. It also contains prebiotics and fiber to support gut and overall health. And there is zero sugar, too. Sweetness comes from stevia and erythritol.

BEST GOAT WHEY PROTEIN
Teraswhey Gluten-Free Certified Goat Whey Protein
Plant-based protein powders aren't your only option if you're sensitive to dairy. Enter goat whey protein. The cold-pressed, non-denatured whey is smooth and creamy, perfect for blending in smoothies.

BEST GRASS-FED WHEY
Promix Grass-Fed Whey Protein Powder
Made from grass-fed cows free of hormones, this protein powder packs in 25 grams of protein and 5.9 grams of BCAAs for ultimate recovery and muscle-building power. It doesn't skimp on flavor either, with multiple tasty options to choose from and subtle sweetness from coconut sugar.

BEST RECOVERY PROTEIN
Ladder Whey Protein Powder
This whey-based protein powder (founded by NBA star Lebron James) has 26g of protein and no artificial sweeteners. What sets it apart is the added tart cherry for enhanced recovery.

BEST UNFLAVORED PROTEIN
KION Clean Protein
This grass-fed whey protein isolate powder boasts 20 grams of high-quality protein per serving and no additives. You won't find any gluten, soy, or sugar on the ingredients list.

Keeping It Regular

Since protein powders are not FDA-regulated, their ingredient lists can be unclear or misleading and sometimes result in gastrointestinal (GI) issues like constipation. Even though protein powders sometimes advertise containing no sugar or being low-carb, a lot of them have artificial sweeteners and sugar alcohols, which can all be linked to stomach upset and diarrhea, says Megan Robinson, RD, a board-certified sports dietitian and running coach.

Robinson also says to keep in mind any intolerances or allergens you might have, especially if you consume protein powders or prepackaged drinks. Whey protein powder, for example, may contain lactose. "And if you have a lactose intolerance, that may be contributing to stomach upset," Robinson says. She suggests looking for protein drinks that are certified by NSF Certified Sport or Informed Choice, two third-party companies that certify protein powders.

The best way to avoid protein-related GI issues is to chow down on high-fiber foods alongside protein sources. Armul recommends prioritizing plant-based proteins (see more page 22). "It's [a] double-whammy. You're getting protein but you're also reaping the benefits of fiber," she says.

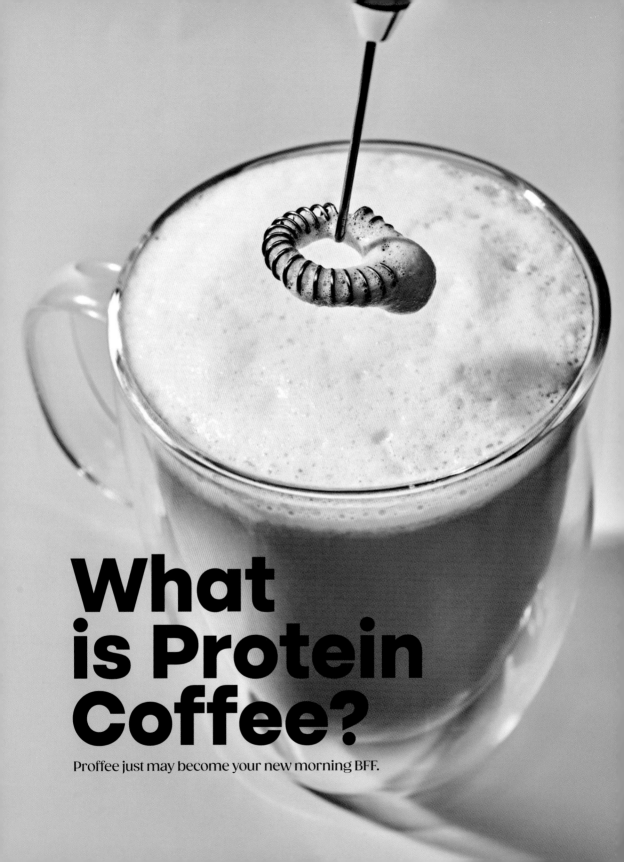

What is Protein Coffee?

Proffee just may become your new morning BFF.

→ **Protein coffee is exactly what it sounds like: adding protein powder or a pre-made shake to your brew. It's super simple and effective. With just one scoop, you're instantly racking up 25 to 30 grams of protein first thing in the morning. Plus, if breakfast has never been your thing anyways, protein coffee or "proffee" is a good way to keep you full and energized until your first meal.**

Of course, you can drink your proffee and enjoy a meal at the same time, too. A scoop of protein powder in your coffee plus two scrambled eggs is around 40 grams of protein! Start the day with a bang!

What are the benefits of protein coffee?

It's the perfect pre-gym boost, for one thing. The caffeine adds that boost of energy, and the protein helps maintain muscle mass and build your tissues and bones. If you just want the protein sans the caffeine, decaf coffee is also is totally fair game, too. Upping your protein before the gym could also help keep your energy levels stable and consistent all day long. Here are a few other great reasons to give it a try:

▶ **It adds more tang to your coffee.**
If you like flavored milks or creamers, using flavored protein powders in your coffee can have the same effect without the added calories, sugar, and fat.

▶ **It can help with weight loss.**
Eating a high-protein breakfast can stabilize blood sugar and prevent glucose spikes better than a high-carb meal, which aids in weight management. Proffee can help with your weight management goals because it keeps your metabolism boosted all day.

Any downsides to protein coffee?

The added protein may change the texture of your drink. Depending on the type of powder you use, your blend may turn out grittier or thicker than you'd like. And, if your protein powder is made with sugar substitutes like stevia, erythritol, or aspartame, you may experience stomach discomfort, bloating, or diarrhea. So, always read the label carefully and choose a powder without artificial sweeteners if they bother you.

How do you make it at home?

Using either a blender or a frother is the ultimate way to thoroughly mix the protein powder into your coffee and get out any clumps. Simply add your preferred milk and a scoop of protein powder and froth until it's fluffy.

Play around with the protein-to-coffee ratio and find what tastes best to you. It really comes down to taste and texture.

Protein coffee works hot or iced, and in fact, the powder blends the easiest when added to cold coffee. It's recommended to blend the hot coffee with protein powder, so it provides a frothy drink.

Bottom line: Customize your proffee to find what tastes best for you and experiment with the flavors, proportions, and temperatures. Want some extra creaminess (and protein, for that matter)? Add a splash of your favorite milk.

What is Protein Water?

Basically water that's been infused with extra protein—typically from a whey-based product, sometimes from collagen. A lot of brands have between 10 and 20 grams of protein, and they are often fruit flavored. There are also powders available that you can add right to your own water, DIY-style! It's a super convenient way to add protein into your diet, and while it may not be enough of a meal or snack on its own, you can, say, pair it with a protein bar for a post-workout recovery snack. Our faves include PWR Lift and Protein2o, and Vital Proteins collagen water.

ANY DOWNSIDES TO PROTEIN WATER?

Check for the amount of sugar or an artificial sweetener in the beverage, and weigh the pros and cons—yes, you could be consuming more protein, but you could also be doing yourself a disservice in another department. Also, don't chug protein right before exercise, as it's slow-digesting and you can risk stomach upset.

Ready, Set, Prep!

If the idea of meal prepping seems intimidating, you're not alone. Trust, some simple steps can make your life a bit easier, especially when prioritizing protein.

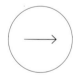

There's nothing worse then the dreaded, "What should I eat?" dilemma around 5 p.m., but meal prepping is an easy solution. Meal prepping allows you to cook on your schedule, so you have homemade, healthy dishes on hand all week.

Plus, meal prepping is a great way to stay on top of your health and fitness goals, says Kelly Jones, RD, sports dietitian and owner of Student Athlete Nutrition.

"Everyone can benefit from meal prepping," she says. But the thought of downing the same salmon, green beans, and quinoa combo four days in a row? Nope, nope, and *nope.* "You don't have to have these lofty goals. You don't have to have a super crazy schedule," Jones explains. "You can just be someone who's looking to do a little bit in advance or take advantage of extra time on the weekend–or whatever day of the week you might have free–to set yourself up for more success later on."

If you don't have time to devote a whole day to cooking, that's okay. There's more than one meal-prep method. "Meal prep can be any level of preparation that you do in advance for the week so that you can make meals and eating snacks easier," says Jones.

Now, there's just the matter of where to start. Follow these smart strategies to help you hit your goals and nix any hangry tendencies.

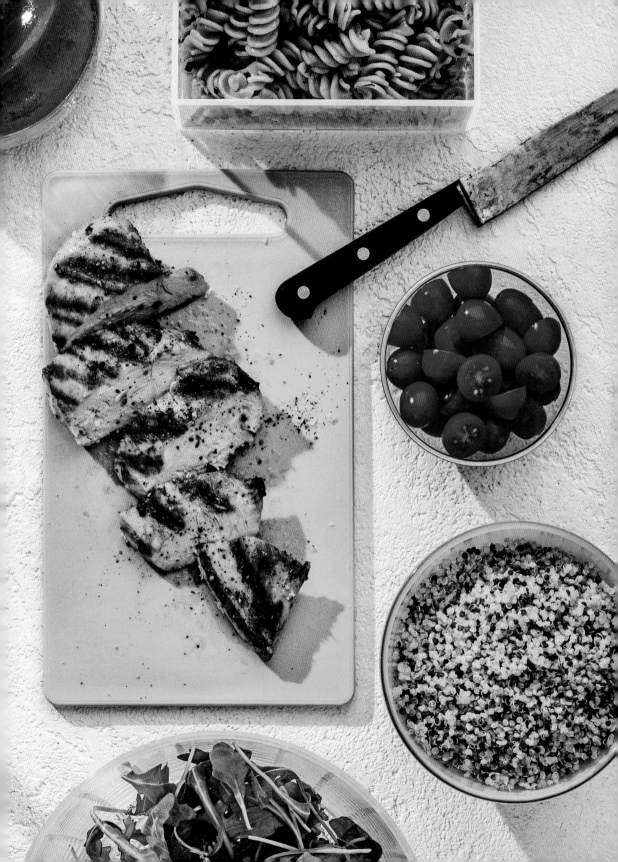

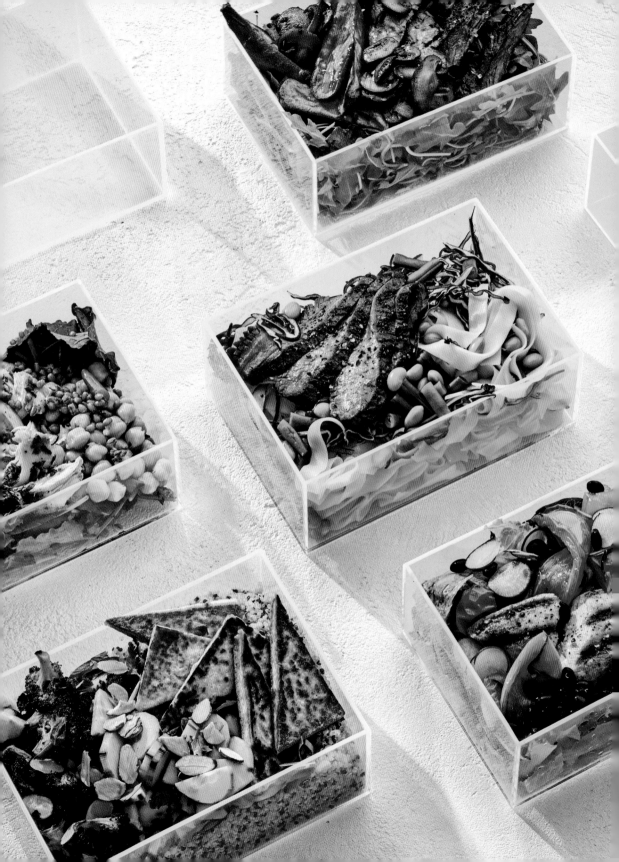

Cook now, eat later.

Have a few extra minutes? Devote some time to cooking up complete meals that you can just grab from the fridge or freezer and reheat at a future date. Or you can spend some time batch-cooking ingredients (like grains) to cut down on prep time later in the week.

Make too much.

If you're already whipping up a recipe, make extra! Most proteins, beans, and grains can easily be doubled to make enough for now and later. Use whatever is left to toss over a salad, stuff into a burrito or wrap, or mix into a grain bowl.

Keep ready-to-eat options on-hand.

Meal prepping doesn't mean you need to prep full meals. Instead, store high-protein, ready-to-eat options like beans, canned tuna, hard-boiled eggs, Greek yogurt, or precooked lentils in your kitchen for easy snacking or add-on ingredients.

Prepare healthy snacks.

When hunger strikes, high-protein snacks are your BFF. Keep simple bites like hard boiled eggs, cut veggies with hummus, or cottage cheese with berries locked and loaded in your fridge.

Invest in good containers.

If your old plastic Tupperware isn't cutting it (a.k.a you can't find any of the proper lids!), invest in new reusable containers. They're sturdy, seal in moisture and flavor, and some are even safe for the fridge, freezer, microwave, and oven.

Switch up the flavors.

Shake things up and get creative with different sauces and flavor profiles to keep grab-and-go ingredients interesting. The *Women's Health* Test Kitchen keeps the sauces and dressings at right on hand for a quick flavor boost.

Super Sauces

● Caper Vinaigrette

Combine 2 shallots, 1/2 cup parsley, 1/4 cup drained capers (all finely chopped), 1 Tbsp lemon zest plus 1/4 cup juice, and 1/2 tsp each salt and pepper, then whisk in 1/2 cup olive oil. Makes about 1 1/2 cups.

● Vegan Caesar

Whisk together 2 tsp lemon zest plus 1/2 cup juice, 1 tsp Dijon mustard, 1 grated clove garlic, and 1 tsp each low-sodium soy sauce and pepper. Whisk in 1 cup olive oil. Makes about 1 1/2 cups.

● Peanut Sauce

In a blender, puree 3/4 cup each creamy all-natural peanut butter and canola oil, 1/2 cup water, 1/4 cup each rice vinegar and fresh lime juice, 1 1/2 Tbsp each low-sodium soy sauce and gochujang, and 2 scallion whites until smooth. Makes about 3 cups.

● Sriracha-Honey Vinaigrette

Whisk together 1/4 cup each cider vinegar and olive oil, 2 Tbsp sriracha, 2 tsp honey, and 1/2 tsp salt. Makes about 2/3 cup.

● Romesco Sauce

In a food processor, pulse 2 cups roasted red peppers (drained), 1 cup flat-leaf parsley, 1/2 cup roasted salted almonds, and a pinch of salt until almost smooth. Makes about 1 3/4 cups.

● Cilantro-Lime Yogurt

In a blender, puree 1 jalapeño (seeded and chopped), 2 cups Greek yogurt, 1 cup cilantro, 1/4 cup fresh lime juice, and 1/2 tsp each ground cumin and salt until smooth. Makes about 2 1/2 cups.

● Mediterranean Olive Sauce

In a blender, puree 2 cups pitted green olives, 1/2 cup olive oil, 1/4 cup lemon juice, 2 tsp Dijon mustard, 1/2 cup flat-leaf parsley, 2 cloves garlic, and 1/4 tsp red pepper flakes until nearly smooth. Makes about 2 1/4 cups.

PART TWO

Protein-Packed Recipes

You certainly know **why protein is important**, but if you are still thinking, "but do I have to eat the same thing every day," the answer is no way. Enter: these delicious options.

Breakfast

Ensure you meet your goals by starting your day right—with an **energizing boost of protein**. These filling a.m. meals—smoothies, eggs, and more—pack a powerful punch.

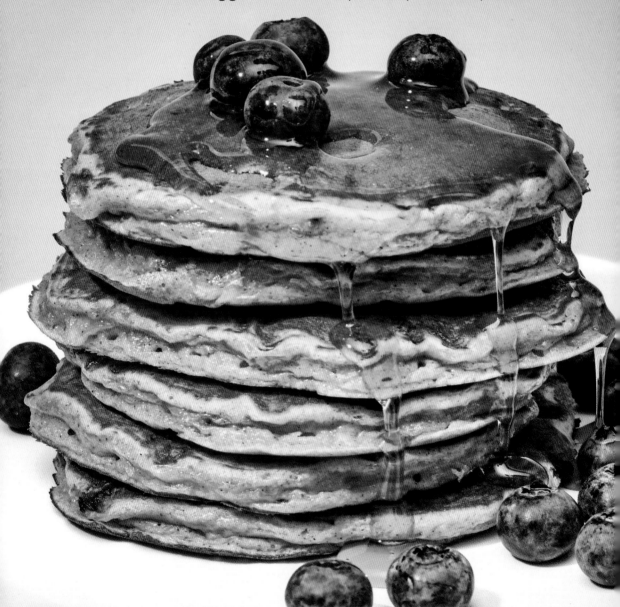

Ultimate Protein Pancakes

TOTAL 25 MIN. **SERVES** 2

- ⅓ cup oat flour
- ¼ cup unflavored whey protein powder
- 1 tsp baking powder
- ¼ tsp ground cinnamon
- Kosher salt
- 1 small ripe banana
- ½ cup low-fat cottage cheese
- 1 large egg
- ½ tsp pure vanilla extract
- Maple syrup and fresh berries, for serving

1. In medium bowl, whisk oat flour, protein powder, baking powder, cinnamon, and pinch of salt.

2. In another medium bowl, mash banana with fork. Whisk in cottage cheese, egg, and vanilla to combine. Gradually add wet ingredients to dry ingredients, whisking just until combined. Let batter rest 5 minutes.

3. Heat large nonstick skillet on medium. Add four scant ¼-cupfuls of batter and flatten into 3½- to 4-inch rounds using side or bottom of measuring cup. Cook until edges are set and bottom is golden brown, 2 to 3 min. Flip and cook until golden brown and cooked through, 1 to 2 min. more. Transfer to plate.

4. Reduce heat to medium-low. Repeat with remaining batter, adjusting heat as necessary. Serve pancakes with maple syrup and berries, if desired.

Per serving (3 pancakes): About 229 calories, 6.5 g fat (2.5 g saturated fat), 114 mg cholesterol, 583 mg sodium, 28 g carbohydrates, 3 g fiber, 9 g sugar (0.5 g added sugar), 17 g protein

POWER UP!
Another great topping for pancakes is creamy Greek yogurt—and ¼ cup adds 6 grams of protein.

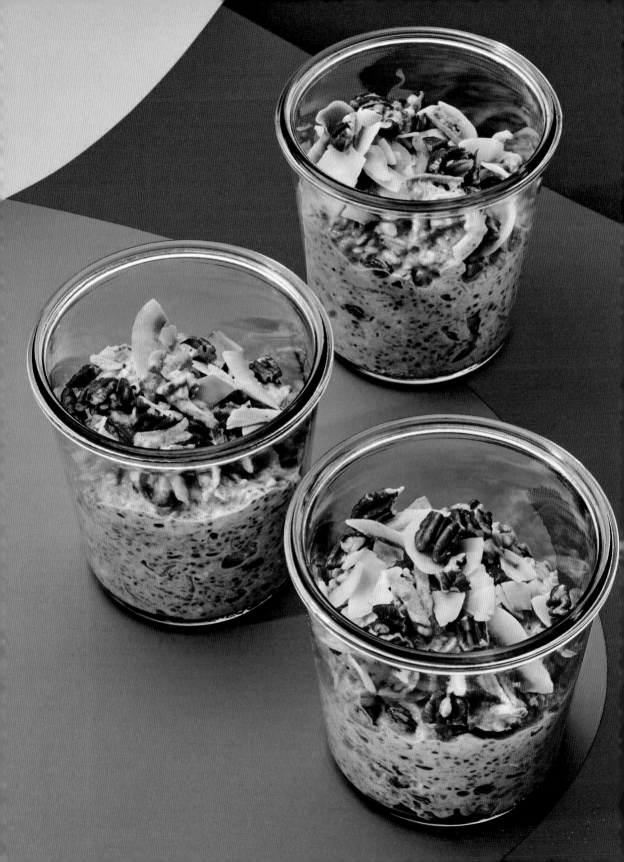

Overnight "Carrot Cake" Oats

TOTAL 10 MIN., PLUS OVERNIGHT COOLING **SERVES** 4 (MAKES 6 CUPS)

2	cups unsweetened soy milk, plus more for thinning
1½	cups whole milk Greek yogurt
3	tsp pure maple syrup
2	tsp ground cinnamon
1½	tsp pure vanilla extract
½	tsp kosher salt
1¼	cups rolled oats
1	large carrot (8 oz), scrubbed and coarsely grated (2½ cups)
⅔	cup toasted pecans, chopped, plus more for topping
½	cup raisins, roughly chopped
¼	cup toasted unsweetened coconut chips, lightly crushed, plus more for topping
¼	cup chia seeds

1. In large bowl, whisk together soy milk, yogurt, maple syrup, cinnamon, vanilla, and salt.

2. Stir in oats, carrot, pecans, raisins, coconut, and chia seeds until well combined. Divide among jars, cover, and refrigerate overnight.

3. Serve, adjusting consistency with additional soy milk as needed. The mixture can be refrigerated for up to 3 days altogether or portioned out. Top just before eating or serving.

Per serving *About 541 calories, 27 g fat (6 g saturated fat), 9 mg cholesterol, 348 mg sodium, 60 g carbohydrates, 13 g fiber, 26.5 g sugar (3 g added sugar), 21 g protein*

Test Kitchen Trick **TRUST US,** stick to rolled oats. Instant oats are the most processed oat variety, and while that cooks quickly for oatmeal, it does not work here. Steel cut oats can be used but they might be a little chewy and dense compared to rolled oats.

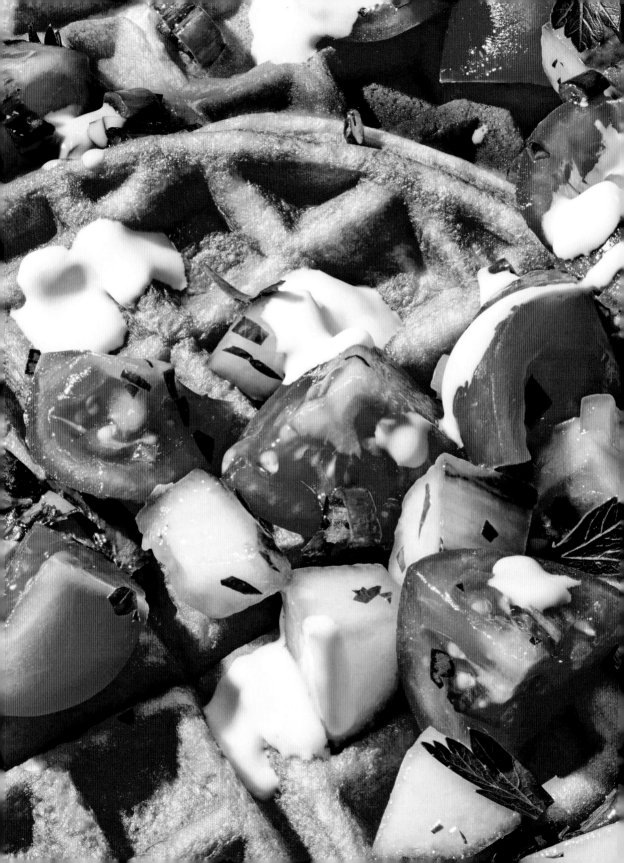

Greek Chickpea Waffles

TOTAL 30 MIN. **SERVES** 4

¾ cup chickpea flour

½ tsp baking soda

½ tsp salt

¾ cup plain 2% Greek yogurt

6 large eggs

Tomatoes, cucumbers, scallion, parsley, yogurt, and lemon juice, for serving

1. Heat oven to 200°F. Set wire rack over rimmed baking sheet and place in oven. Heat waffle iron per directions.

2. In large bowl, whisk together flour, baking soda, and salt. In small bowl, whisk together yogurt and eggs. Stir wet ingredients into dry ingredients.

3. Lightly coat waffle iron with nonstick cooking spray and, in batches, drop ¼ to ½ cup batter into each section of iron and cook until golden brown, 4 to 5 min. Transfer to oven and keep warm. Repeat with remaining batter.

4. Serve topped with tomatoes, cucumbers, and scallion tossed with salt, pepper, and parsley. Drizzle with yogurt mixed with lemon juice.

Per serving *About 272 calories, 12.5 g fat (4 g saturated fat), 277 mg cholesterol, 573 mg sodium, 16 g carbohydrates, 2 g fiber, 5 g sugars (0 g added sugars), 22 g protein*

FIBER FIX

Chickpea flour is full of protein and fiber too. A great thickening agent, you can use it as a substitute for all-purpose flour in savory dishes like soups or stews or to bind ingredients like meatballs.

Spiced Blueberry Smoothie Bowl

TOTAL 5 MIN. **SERVES** 1

1 cup frozen blueberries

1 banana, sliced and frozen

½ cup frozen cauliflower

½ cup unsweetened almond milk, plus more as needed

3 Tbsp unsweetened pea protein (vanilla or regular)

1 tsp flaxseed

¼ tsp ground cinnamon

⅛ tsp ground ginger

Fresh berries and buckwheat granola, for serving

In blender, puree all ingredients until smooth (mixture will be thick), adding more almond milk a little at a time as necessary to adjust consistency. Transfer to bowl and top with fresh berries and buckwheat granola.

Per serving *About 325 calories, 5.5 g fat (1 g saturated fat), 0 mg cholesterol, 357 mg sodium, 52 g carbohydrates, 10 g fiber, 29 g sugars (0 g added sugars), 22 g protein*

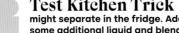

Test Kitchen Trick **IF YOU PREP** this smoothie ahead of serving it might separate in the fridge. Add it back to a blender with a few cubes of ice or some additional liquid and blend until it's the consistency you want.

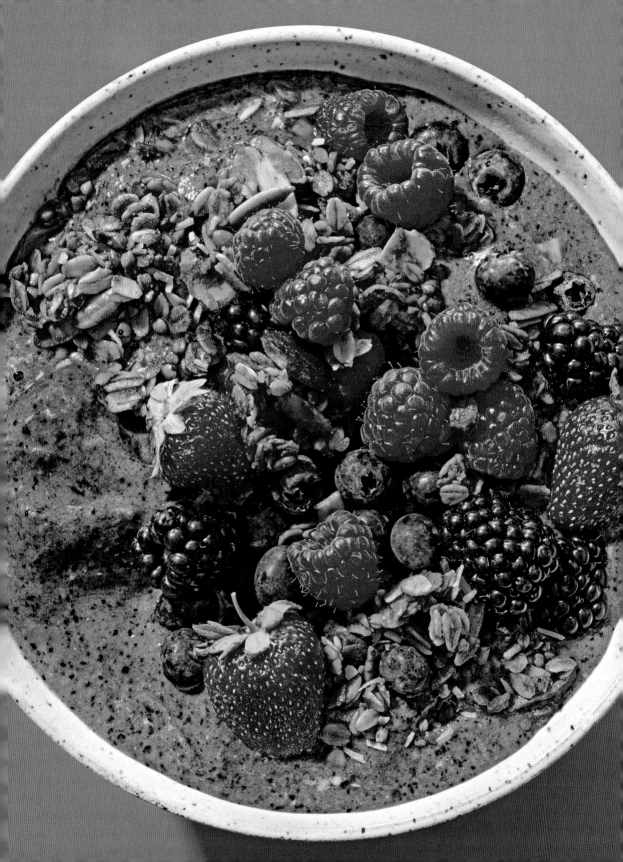

Chocolate Berry Protein Smoothie

TOTAL 5 MIN. **SERVES** 1

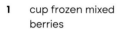

1	cup frozen mixed berries
1	cup baby spinach
1	scoop chocolate protein powder
1	Tbsp unsalted sunflower seeds
	Pinch of kosher salt
¾	cup water

In blender, puree all ingredients until smooth and creamy and serve.

Per serving 261 calories, 8 g fat (1.5 g saturated), 0 mg cholesterol, 450 mg sodium, 24 g carbohydrates, 9 g fiber, 10.5 g sugar (0 g added sugar), 24 g protein

Tropical Green Protein Smoothie

TOTAL 5 MIN. **SERVES** 1

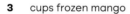

3	cups frozen mango
1	cup frozen peas
1	cup baby spinach
1	scoop vanilla protein powder
1	Tbsp lightly salted cashews
	Pinch of lime zest
¾	cup coconut water

In blender, puree all ingredients until smooth and creamy and serve.

Per serving About 537 calories, 7 g fat (2 g saturated fat), 0 mg cholesterol, 460 mg sodium, 106 g carbohydrates, 16 g fiber, 78 g sugar (3 g added sugar), 24 g protein

 Prep Ahead **FREEZE ALL** ingredients but coconut water in a jar. When ready, blend with coconut water and serve in the same jar—no extra dishes!

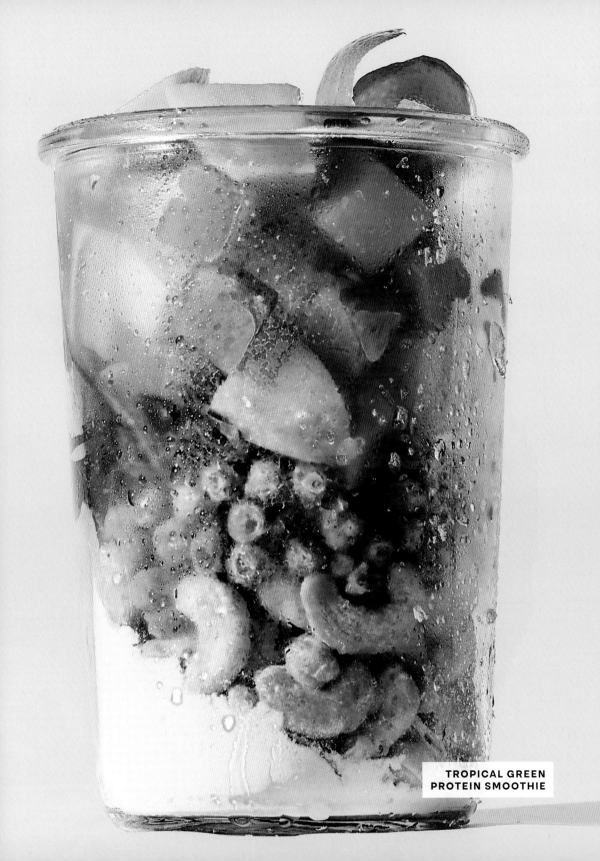

TROPICAL GREEN
PROTEIN SMOOTHIE

Avocado Spinach Green Smoothie

TOTAL 10 MIN. **SERVES** 1

2	cups spinach, thick stems discarded
⅔	cup water
½	cup kefir
½	tsp lemon zest plus 1 tsp juice
1	large avocado
1	½-inch piece fresh ginger, sliced
2	Tbsp cilantro
1	scoop collagen
Pinch of kosher salt	
¼	English cucumber, cut into half-moons and frozen
1	cup seedless green grapes, frozen

In blender, puree all ingredients until smooth and creamy and serve.

Per serving About 259 calories, 6 g fat (1.5 g saturated fat), 7 mg cholesterol, 212 mg sodium, 43 g carbohydrates, 35.5 g sugars (0 g added sugars), 6 g fiber, 18 g protein

POWER UP!
Pick any yogurt you like for your smoothie—Greek, goat's milk, soy, coconut, or plain—to amp up protein power.

Green Machine Smoothie

TOTAL 5 MIN. **SERVES** 1

½	cup nondairy coconut yogurt
2	cups spinach
1½	cups frozen pineapple chunks
¼	cup frozen peas

In blender, puree all ingredients until smooth and creamy and serve.

Per serving About 321 calories, 8 g fat (6.5 g saturated fat), 7 g protein, 58 mg sodium, 60 g carbohydrates, 16.5 g sugars (0 g added sugars), 10 g fiber

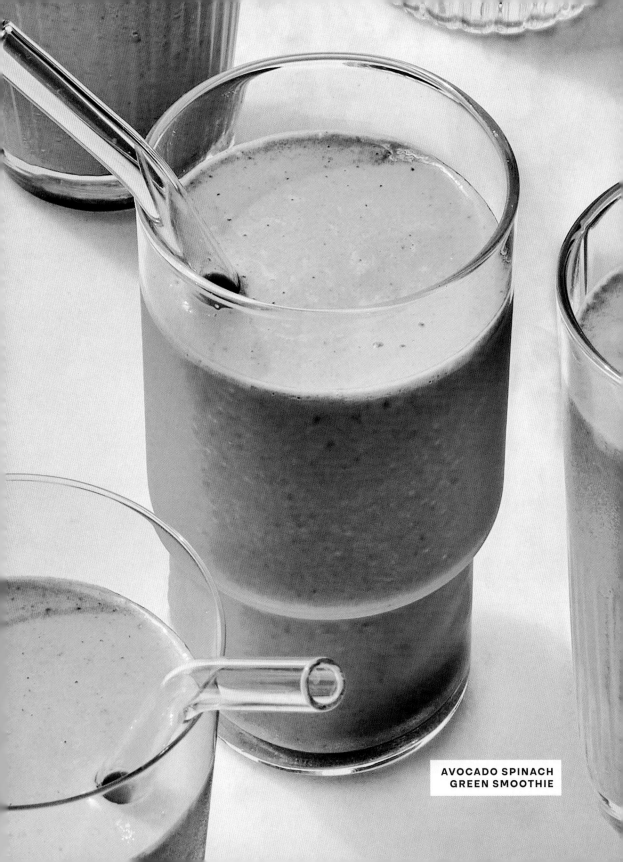

AVOCADO SPINACH
GREEN SMOOTHIE

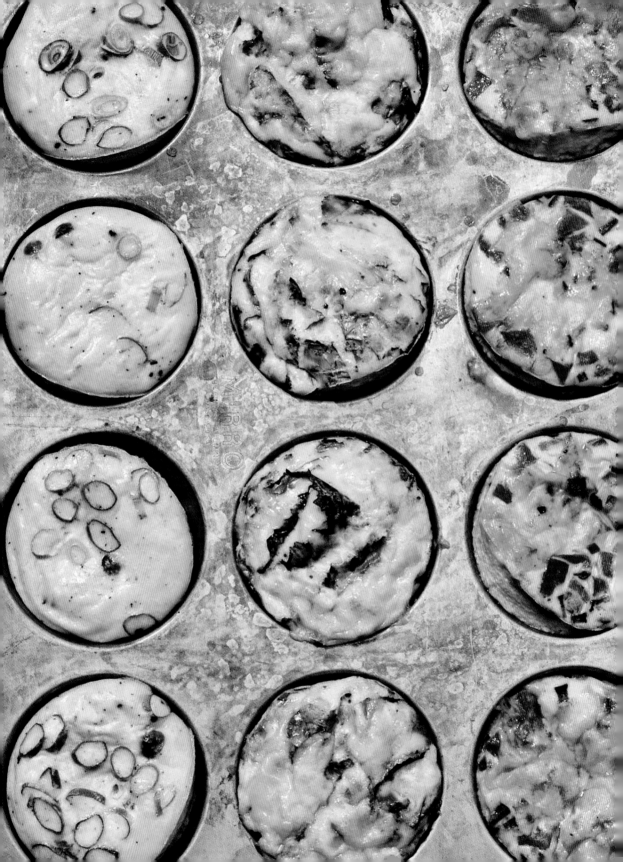

Meal Prep Egg Bites

TOTAL 35 MIN. SERVES 12

BASIC EGG BITES

Nonstick cooking spray

8 large eggs

1 cup milk

Kosher salt and pepper

SWEET PEA
AND RICOTTA

3 Tbsp ricotta

¾ cup frozen peas,
thawed and
coarsely mashed

4 scallions,
thinly sliced

PICO AND CHEDDAR

1¼ cup pico de gallo,
drained well

3 oz extra-sharp
Cheddar, coarsely
grated (about 1 cup)

GREENS AND GRUYÈRE

2 cups baby kale,
roughly chopped

3 oz Gruyère, coarsely
grated (about 1 cup)

1. Heat oven to 350°F. Coat 12-cup muffin pan with nonstick cooking spray.

2. In large bowl, whisk together eggs, milk, ½ tsp each salt and pepper and ricotta, if using. Divide half of egg mixture among prepared muffin cups, followed by desired fillings (except grated cheese) and then remaining egg mixture. Top with grated cheese, if using. Bake until puffed and set, 20 to 25 min.

Basic Egg Bites (per serving) *About 61 calories, 4 g fat (1.5 g saturated fat), 126 mg cholesterol, 140 mg sodium, 2 g carbohydrates, 0 g fiber, 1 g sugar (0 g added sugar), 5 g protein*

Sweet Pea and Ricotta (per serving) *About 76 calories, 4 g fat (1.5 g saturated fat), 128 mg cholesterol, 144 mg sodium, 3 g carbohydrates, 1 g fiber, 2 g sugar (0 g added sugar), 6 g protein*

Pico and Cheddar (per serving) *About 100 calories, 6 g fat (3 g saturated fat), 136 mg cholesterol, 308 mg sodium, 4 g carbohydrates, 0 g fiber, 3 g sugar (0 g added sugar), 7 g protein*

Greens and Gruyère (per serving) *About 92 calories, 6 g fat (2.5 g saturated fat), 134 mg cholesterol, 194 mg sodium, 2 g carbohydrates, 0 g fiber, 1 g sugar (0 g added sugar), 7 g protein*

Prep Ahead **WRAP EACH** egg bite in plastic and freeze up to 1 month. To reheat, remove plastic wrap and microwave each muffin, wrapped in damp paper towel, until warmed through, about 2 min.

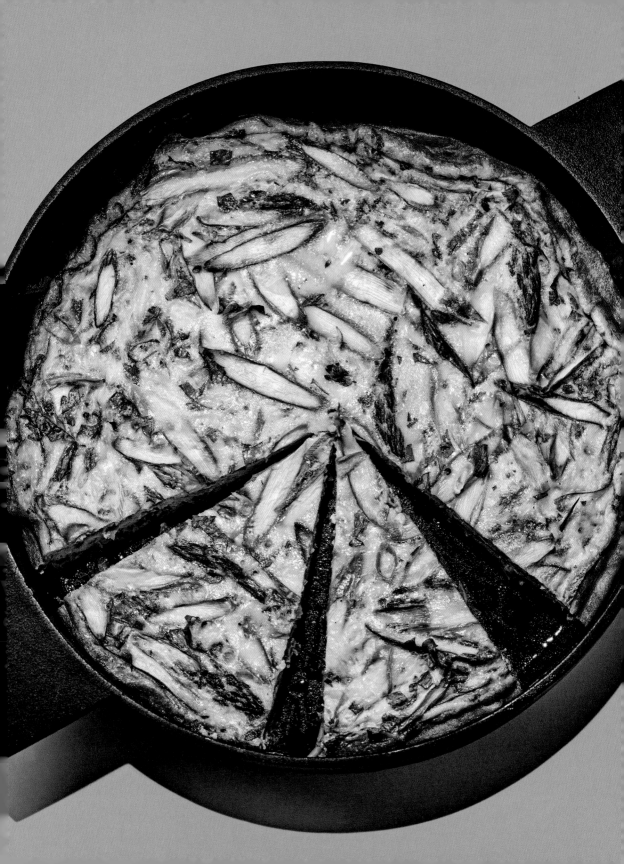

Asparagus and Scallion Frittata

TOTAL 20 MIN. **SERVES** 4

1½ tsp olive oil

1 lb asparagus,
   trimmed and cut into
   1-inch pieces on bias

Kosher salt and pepper

4 scallions, thinly
   sliced, white
   and green parts
   separated

8 large eggs

2 Tbsp sour cream

1 tsp Dijon mustard

½ cup flat-leaf
   parsley, chopped

2 oz Gruyère, grated

Mixed green salad,
for serving

1. Heat oven to 425°F. In 9- to 10-inch cast-iron skillet on medium, heat oil. Add asparagus, season with ¼ tsp each salt and pepper; sauté 2 min. Add scallion whites and cook, tossing, 1 min. Remove from heat.

2. Meanwhile, in bowl, whisk together eggs, sour cream, mustard, and pinch each of salt and pepper. Fold in scallion greens, parsley, and cheese.

3. Add egg mixture to pan and cook until edges have begun to set, about 2 min. Transfer skillet to oven; bake until center is just set, 8 to 10 min. Serve with green salad, if desired.

Per serving About 280 calories, 20.5 g fat (7 g saturated fat), 391 mg cholesterol, 438 mg sodium, 5 g carbohydrates, 2 g fiber, 2 g sugar (0 g added sugars), 19 g protein

Test Kitchen Trick **WHEN PREPARING** the egg mixture, beat until combined but don't keep going! Overbeating eggs can introduce too much air to the mixture and cause the frittata to expand while in the oven and deflate and be dry once cooled.

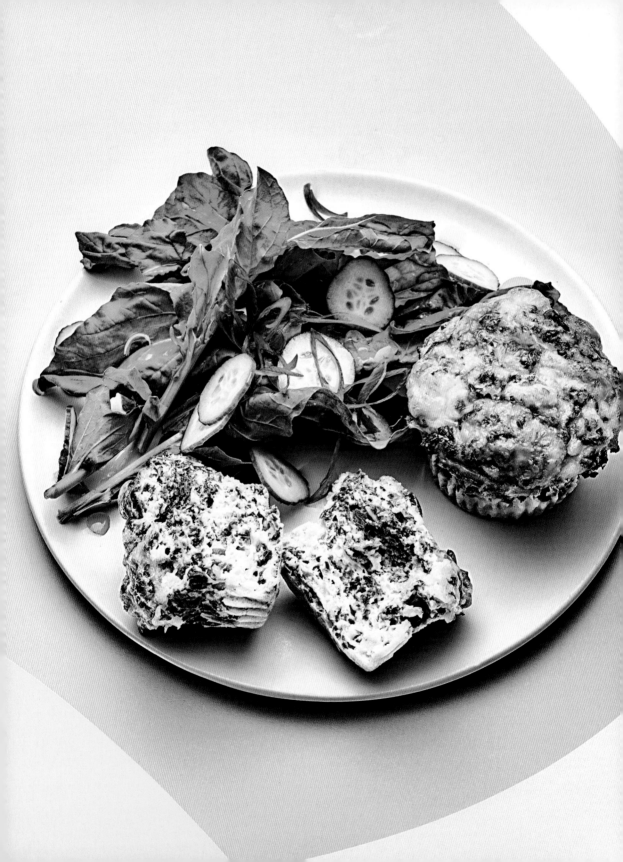

Spinach and Cottage Cheese Spoonbread Muffins

TOTAL 40 MIN., PLUS COOLING **SERVES** 6 (MAKES 12 MUFFINS)

Canola oil spray,
for greasing

6 Tbsp finely ground
yellow cornmeal

¾ tsp baking powder

½ tsp kosher salt

½ tsp pepper

½ tsp freshly grated
nutmeg (optional)

6 large eggs

1½ cups lowfat
cottage cheese

4 oz Gruyère cheese,
coarsely grated
(1½ cups), divided

4 scallions,
thinly sliced

1 16-oz bag frozen
chopped spinach,
thawed and
squeezed very well

1. Heat oven to 475°F. Line 12-cup muffin pan
with foil liners and coat with canola oil spray.
2. In small bowl, whisk together cornmeal, baking
powder, salt, pepper, and nutmeg (if using).
3. In large bowl, whisk eggs then stir in cottage
cheese and 1¼ cups Gruyère. Stir in scallions,
spinach, then dry ingredients. Divide among
prepared liners (about ⅓ cup each) then
sprinkle with remaining Gruyère.
4. Bake until golden brown and puffy, 16 to 18 min.
Let cool 5 min. before serving.

Per serving *About 250 calories, 13 g fat (6 g saturated fat),*
214 mg cholesterol, 676 mg sodium, 13 g carbohydrates,
4g fiber, 3.5 g sugar (0 g added sugar), 22 g protien

Prep Ahead **TO STORE MUFFINS,** let cool completely on wire rack.
Refrigerate in airtight container or resealable bag separated with pieces
of parchment up to 5 days or freeze up to 2 months. To reheat: Remove
parchment and foil liners and wrap 2 muffins in damp paper towel; microwave
until heated through, 30 to 45 sec. from fridge or 1 min. from freezer.

Breakfast Burritos

TOTAL 15 MIN. **SERVES** 4

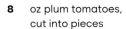

8	oz plum tomatoes, cut into pieces
¼	red onion, roughly chopped
½	small red chile, seeded if desired
¼	cup cilantro, plus more for serving
	Kosher salt
6	large eggs
2	tsp olive oil
3	oz extra-sharp Cheddar, coarsely grated (about 1 cup), divided
4	large flour tortillas, warmed
¾	cup refried beans
2	scallions, thinly sliced

1. In blender, puree tomatoes, onion, chile, cilantro, and ¼ tsp salt. Transfer to skillet and simmer until thickened, about 8 min.

2. Beat eggs with 1 Tbsp water and ¼ tsp salt. Heat oil in medium skillet on medium and scramble eggs to desired doneness; fold in ½ cup cheddar.

3. Spread tortillas with beans (3 Tbsp each), then top with eggs and remaining ½ cup Cheddar. Spoon 2 Tbsp salsa on each, then sprinkle with scallions. Roll burritos, folding sides over filling and rolling from bottom up.

4, If desired, crisp both sides of burrito in nonstick skillet on medium. Serve with any remaining salsa and cilantro.

Per serving *About 467 calories, 22.5 g fat (9.5 g saturated fat), 302 mg cholesterol, 1,251 mg sodium, 44 g carbohydrates, 4 g fiber, 4.5 g sugar (0 g added sugar), 24 g protein*

Prep Ahead **FYI: You can freeze foil-wrapped burritos up to three (!) weeks. To reheat, remove foil and microwave, flipping once, until heated through, three to five min.**

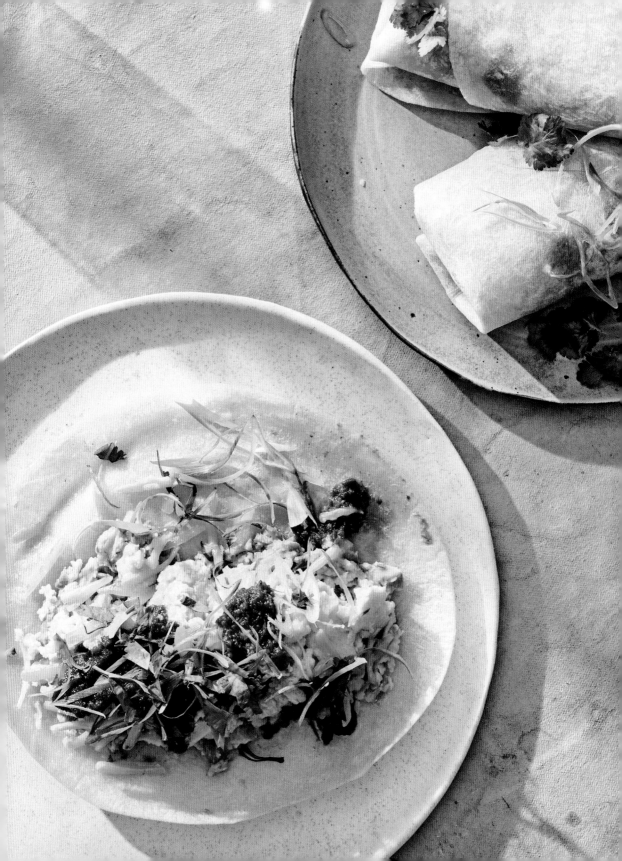

Sheet Pan Egg Tacos

TOTAL 20 MIN. **SERVES** 4

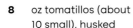

8 oz tomatillos (about 10 small), husked

1 jalapeño, halved and seeded

1 Tbsp olive oil

Kosher salt

8 small corn tortillas

4 oz sharp Cheddar, coarsely grated

8 large eggs

2 cups fresh cilantro, plus more for serving

2 Tbsp fresh lime juice

Sliced radishes, for serving

1. Arrange one oven rack 6 inches from broiler and another about 12 inches from broiler; heat broiler. On rimmed baking sheet, toss tomatillos, jalapeño, oil, and pinch of salt. Broil on top rack until tender and charred in spots, 8 to 10 min. Transfer to blender.

2. Meanwhile, place tortillas on second baking sheet. Divide cheese among tortillas, leaving slight well in center; place an egg in each well. Broil on middle rack to desired doneness, 4 to 6 min. for runny yolks.

3, Add cilantro, lime juice, and ¼ tsp salt to blender and puree until smooth. Serve salsa verde with tacos; top with radishes and cilantro if desired.

Per serving *About 433 calories, 28 g fat (13 g saturated fat), 410 mg cholesterol, 559 mg sodium, 22 g carbohydrates, 5 g fiber, 5 g sugar (0 g added sugar), 25 g protein*

> **"The one food that is high in protein that I do not miss is eggs in the morning for breakfast. Any kind of eggs, I eat them all."**
>
> *Sue Bird, four-time WNBA champion, five-time Olympic gold medalist*

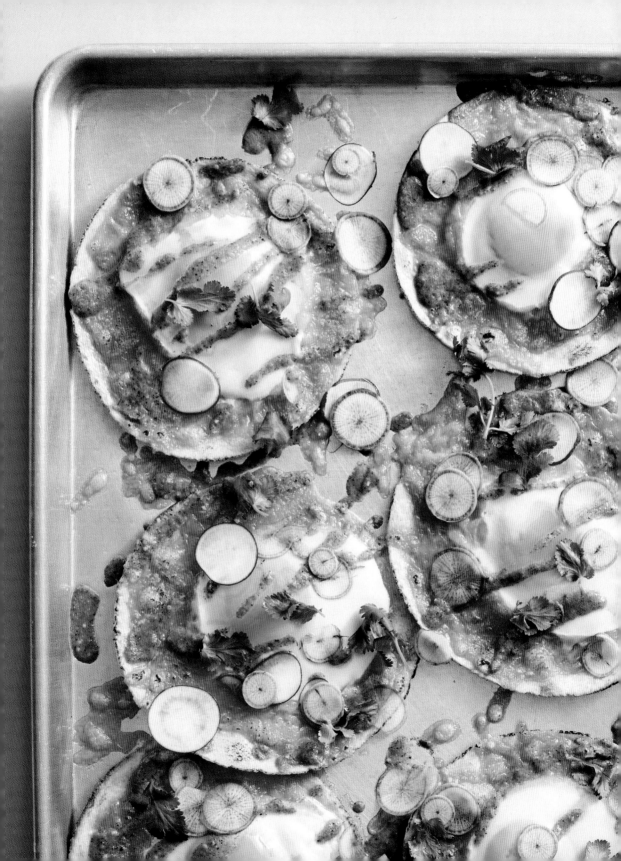

Buckwheat Breakfast Salad

TOTAL 30 MIN. **SERVES** 4

1	cup buckwheat groats, divided
¼	tsp smoked paprika
3	Tbsp olive oil, divided
	Kosher salt and pepper
8	large eggs
1	Tbsp sherry vinegar
1	tsp country-style Dijon mustard
½	tsp honey
4	small heads Little Gem or oak leaf lettuce (8 oz total), trimmed and leaves separated
1	small head frisée (about 4 oz), trimmed and torn into pieces
2	oz aged Gouda, shaved with vegetable peeler
	Flaky salt and cracked pepper, for serving

1. Heat oven to 300°F. On small, rimmed baking sheet, toss ½ cup groats with smoked paprika, 1 Tbsp oil, and ⅛ tsp each kosher salt and pepper. Spread in even layer and bake, stirring halfway through, until golden brown, 25 to 30 min. Let cool.

2. Meanwhile, cook remaining ½ cup groats per package directions; set aside.

3. Bring medium saucepan of water to a boil and fill bowl with ice water. Add eggs and rapidly simmer, 6 min. for jammy eggs, then immediately transfer to prepared ice water to stop the cooking. When cool enough to handle, drain and peel eggs.

4. Meanwhile, in large bowl, whisk together vinegar, mustard, honey, and ¼ tsp each kosher salt and pepper. Slowly whisk in remaining 2 Tbsps oil until fully incorporated. Toss with lettuce and frisée to coat. Divide among bowls. Top with cooked buckwheat, soft-boiled eggs (halved lengthwise), Gouda, toasted buckwheat, and flaky salt and cracked pepper, if desired.

Per serving *About 460 calories, 27 g fat (8 g saturated fat), 429 mg cholesterol, 499 mg sodium, 35 g carbohydrates, 6 g fiber, 1.5 g sugar (0.5 g added sugar), 22 g protein*

POWER UP!
Buckwheat is a superfood seed that's packed with many nutrients like fiber, which aids in digestion. Plus, it's a complete plant protein and naturally gluten-free.

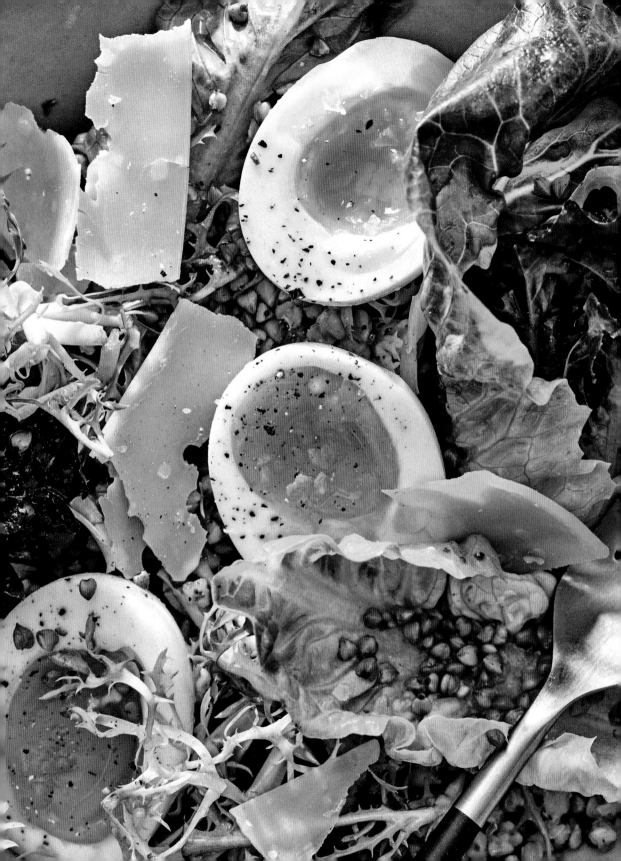

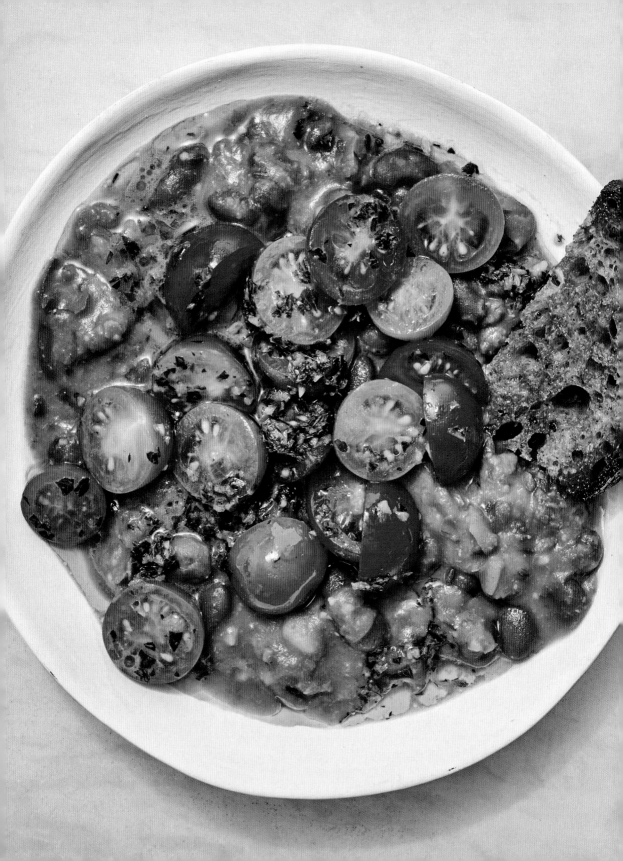

Medames-Style Fava Beans

TOTAL 20 MIN. **SERVES** 4

2	tsp cumin seeds
1	15-oz can fava beans, drained
1	15-oz can red kidney beans, drained
3	cloves garlic
½	jalapeño, roughly chopped
1	cup parsley leaves, packed
¼	cup lemon juice
	Kosher salt
¼	cup extra-virgin olive oil
12	oz multicolored cherry tomatoes, quartered and halved
4	pieces whole-grain bread, toasted and cut into triangles, if desired

1. In medium saucepan on medium, toast cumin seeds, 45 seconds. Remove from heat, add beans and ¼ cup water, and roughly mash. Cook until heated through, 3 min. Adjust consistency with additional water as necessary, so mixture is thick and saucy.
2. In food processor, finely chop garlic and jalapeño. Add parsley and pulse to finely chop. Pulse in lemon juice and ¼ tsp salt to combine. Add oil and pulse once (mixture should not be emulsified); transfer to bowl.
3. Fold tomatoes into parsley sauce. Serve tomatoes spooned over warm fava mixture, with toast if desired.

Per serving *434 calories, 16.5 g fat (2.5 g saturated fat), 5 mg cholesterol, 939 mg sodium, 54 g carbohydrates, 14 g fiber, 3.5 g sugars (0 g added sugars), 20 g protein*

Prep Ahead **MEDAMES** is a hearty Egyptian fava bean stew often served for breakfast but it can also be a protein-packed side for lunch or dinner.

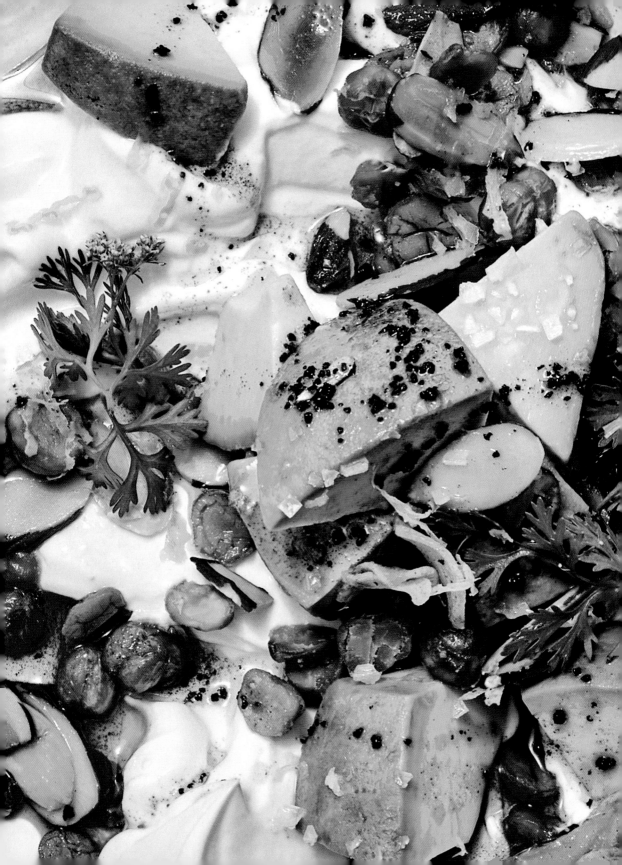

Yogurt with Avocado and Chickpea "Granola"

TOTAL 20 MIN. **SERVES** 4

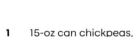

1   15-oz can chickpeas, rinsed and roughly chopped

6   Tbsp olive oil, divided

⅓   cup sliced almonds

2   tsp coriander seeds, crushed

2   cloves garlic, thinly sliced

½   tsp sumac

¼   tsp smoked paprika

1½ cups plain Greek yogurt

1   large avocado, sliced

Kosher salt and lemon zest, for serving

1. Heat oven to 400°F. On rimmed baking sheet, toss chickpeas with 1 Tbsp oil; roast 20 min. Toss with almonds and coriander and roast until chickpeas are crisp and almonds are golden, about 5 min. more.
2. Meanwhile, heat remaining oil and garlic in small saucepan on low and cook, stirring occasionally, until golden brown, 3 to 4 min. Remove from heat and stir in sumac and smoked paprika; let cool.
3. Divide yogurt and avocado among plates. Top with chickpea granola, then spoon garlic and oil on top. Sprinkle with pinch of salt and grated lemon zest.

Per serving About 514 calories, 40 g fat (7 g saturated fat), 4 mg cholesterol, 218 mg sodium, 27 g carbohydrates, 10 g fiber, 7.5 g sugars (0 g added sugars), 16 g protein

POWER UP!
Adding a sprinkle of your favorite nuts to salads, parfaits, or even toast gives a protein boost.

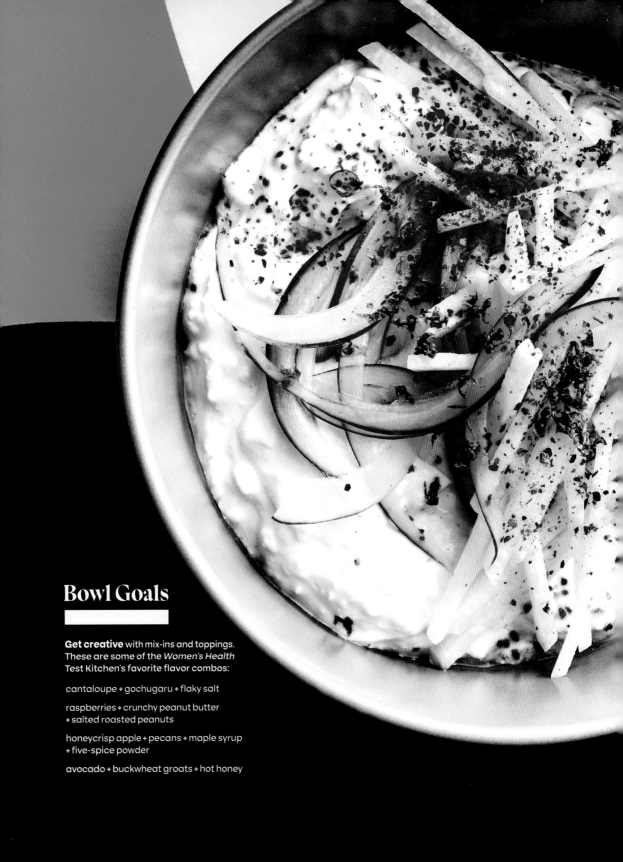

Bowl Goals

Get creative with mix-ins and toppings. These are some of the *Women's Health* Test Kitchen's favorite flavor combos:

cantaloupe + gochugaru + flaky salt

raspberries + crunchy peanut butter + salted roasted peanuts

honeycrisp apple + pecans + maple syrup + five-spice powder

avocado + buckwheat groats + hot honey

Jicama and Tajín Cottage Cheese

TOTAL 30 MIN. **SERVES** 4

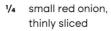

¼ small red onion, thinly sliced

½ tsp lime zest plus 1 Tbsp lime juice

½ cup lowfat cottage cheese

½ cup 2% Greek yogurt

½ small jicama, cut into matchsticks (¼ cup)

Tajín, for sprinkling

In small bowl, combine onion and lime juice, let sit 5 min. In another small bowl, stir together cottage cheese and yogurt. Top with jicama, onion, and lime zest. Sprinkle with Tajín.

Per serving *About 206 calories, 5 g fat (3 g saturated fat), 26 mg cholesterol, 481 mg sodium, 16 g carbohydrates, 2 g fiber, 10.5 g sugar (0 g added sugar), 25 g protein*

Prep Ahead **TRIPLE OR QUADRUPLE** the base recipe, portion out if desired, and refrigerate up to 5 days. When ready to serve, top as desired (we also like: celery, pickle, and dill or other combos at left).

Avocado and Sardine Toast

TOTAL 5 MIN. **SERVES** 4

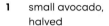

1 small avocado, halved

2 thick slices sourdough bread, toasted

1 lemon

Kosher salt

½ 3.75- to 4.5-oz. can sardines, drained, halved

Red pepper flakes

Scoop avocado out onto toast and mash. Zest lemon over it and sprinkle with pinch of salt. Top with sardines and sprinkle with red pepper flakes.

Per serving *About 589 calories, 31.5 g fat (6.5 g saturated fat), 0 mg cholesterol, 865 mg sodium, 57 g carbohydrates, 12 g fiber, 5 g sugars (0 g added sugars), 24 g protein*

> **When I know my day is going to be slammed, this toast is my morning prescription for an extra hit of energy as soon as possible.”**
>
> *Kat Gordon, owner, Muddy's Bake Shop, Memphis*

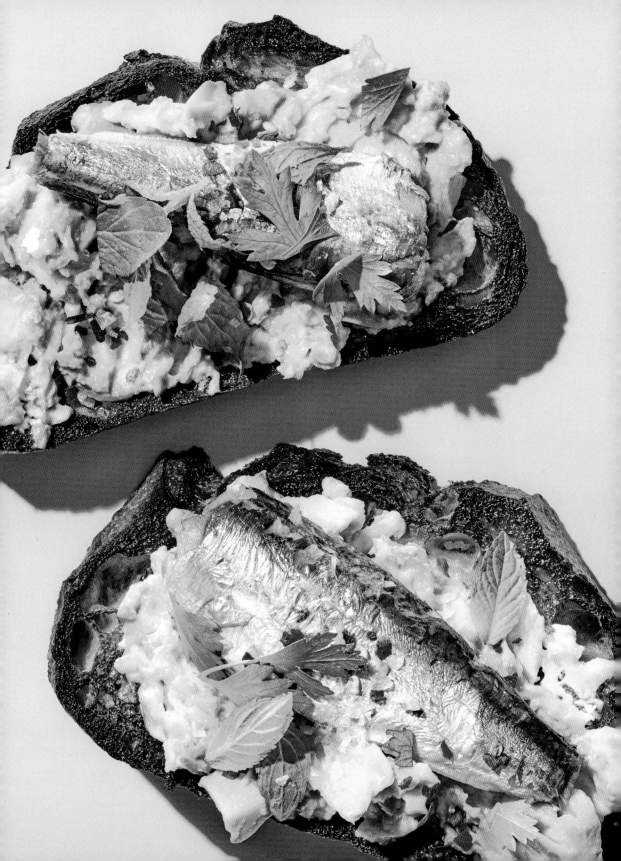

Seeded Buckwheat Pancakes with Smoked Salmon

TOTAL 25 MIN. **SERVES** 4

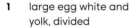

1 large egg white and yolk, divided

⅔ cup cashew milk or milk of choice

½ cup buckwheat flour

Kosher salt and black pepper

3 Tbsp toasted sunflower seeds

3 Tbsp toasted sesame seeds

2 tsp avocado oil

½ cup Greek yogurt

½ small red onion, very thinly sliced

8 oz smoked salmon

¼ cup dill

Lemon wedges, for serving

1. In medium bowl, whisk together egg yolk and cashew milk. Stir in flour and pinch each of salt and pepper until just combined.

2. In second bowl, beat egg white until soft peaks form. Fold into buckwheat mixture, along with sunflower and sesame seeds, until just combined.

3. Rub 1 tsp oil in large nonstick skillet, then heat on medium. In batches, cook ¼-cupfuls until nearly set and bottoms are golden brown, about 3 min. Flip and cook until just cooked through, 1 min. more. Transfer to plate and cover to keep warm. Repeat with remaining batter, adding more oil as necessary.

4. Serve, topped with yogurt, onion, smoked salmon, dill, additional black pepper, and lemon wedges.

Per serving *About 278 calories, 15 g fat (2.5 g saturated fat), 43 mg cholesterol, 477 mg sodium, 16 g carbohydrates, 3 g fiber, 2.5 g sugars (0 g added sugars), 20 g protein*

FIBER FIX
"Fiber gives your digestive system a little extra love," says Yasi Ansari, RD, national media spokesperson for the Academy of Nutrition and Dietetics.

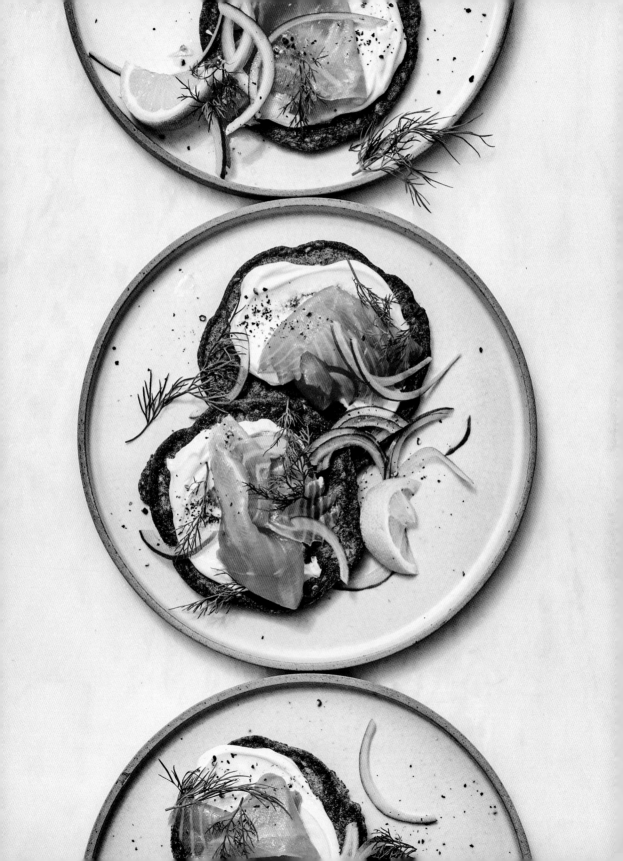

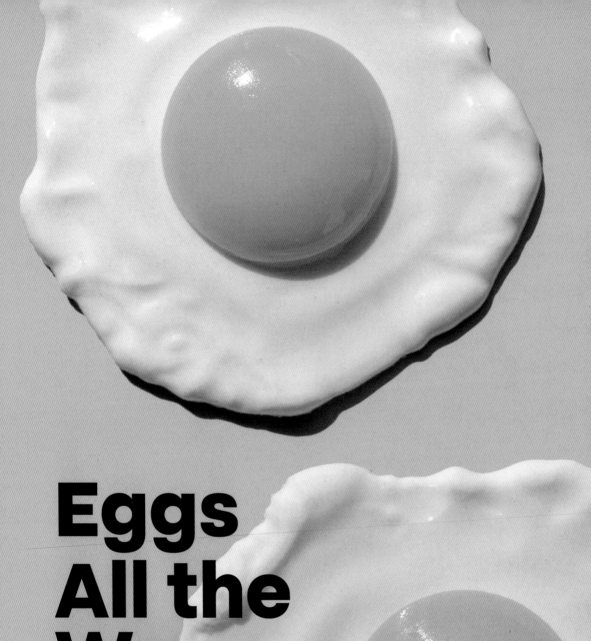

Eggs
All the
Way

Next time you are standing in
front of the stove thinking
"What do I do next?" turn to this
ultimate cooking cheat sheet.

Ah, the almighty egg. A breakfast staple that deserves all of its glory. Not only are eggs the gold standard when it comes to protein (seriously, they are considered a perfect protein source), they can help set you up for a better day of eating overall.

Participants who consumed eggs for breakfast felt fuller and more satisfied for longer compared to those who had cereal and orange juice, according to a small study in the *International Journal of Environmental Research and Public Health*.

The next time you want an egg (or three), follow these cooking instructions.

Scrambled
In large bowl, whisk together 8 large eggs, 1 Tbsp water, and ½ tsp each kosher salt and pepper. Heat 1 Tbsp olive oil or unsalted butter in 10-inch nonstick skillet on medium. Add eggs and cook, stirring with rubber spatula every few seconds, to desired doneness, 2 to 3 min. for medium-soft eggs. Serves 4.

Fried (Over Easy)
Heat nonstick skillet on medium with oil lightly coating bottom. Crack eggs in and cook until bottom is set, about 1 min., then slide spatula under each egg, and with a quick flip, turn over (don't lift too high, or you might break the yolk); cook until whites are set, about 1 min. more.

Sunny-Side Up
Heat nonstick skillet on medium with oil lightly coating bottom. Crack eggs in and cook until tops of whites are set but yolks are still runny, about 3 min. Remove pan from heat and use spatula to transfer to plates. (Tip: You can use a spatula to spread out runnier part of the albumen, a.k.a. egg white.)

Hard-Boiled
Bring medium saucepan of water to a boil. Using large, slotted spoon, gently lower eggs into boiling water. Simmer for 6 min. for jammy, medium-cooked eggs or 11 min. for hard-boiled eggs with yolks cooked all the way through. If you prefer yolks somewhere in the middle, experiment with 7-, 8-, or 9-minute eggs to find your perfect level of doneness. Cool in ice bath (this prevents them from overcooking and makes them easier to peel) and let sit until shells are cool to the touch. Peel and eat or refrigerate in shells for up to a week.

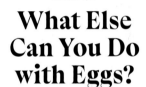

What Else Can You Do with Eggs?

This humble a.m. staple is actually an underrated all-star for other meals too.

TOP OFF GREENS
Move aside, Parm. Grating a hard-boiled egg over roasted asparagus, blanched green beans, or a simple salad adds richness (plus a few extra nutrients, like vitamin A and lutein) and can turn your go-to side into a whole filling meal. (Go for a coarse grater to create bigger pieces of egg.

USE AS A SUPER SAUCE
Go beyond toast and top a bowl of spaghetti with a sunny-side-up egg (the runny yolk becomes a built-in pasta sauce!).

BUMP UP YOUR BROTH
Add whisked whole eggs to simmering stock to build body and give ordinary soup a luxe feel—think eggdrop or lemony avgolemono, a Greek favorite.

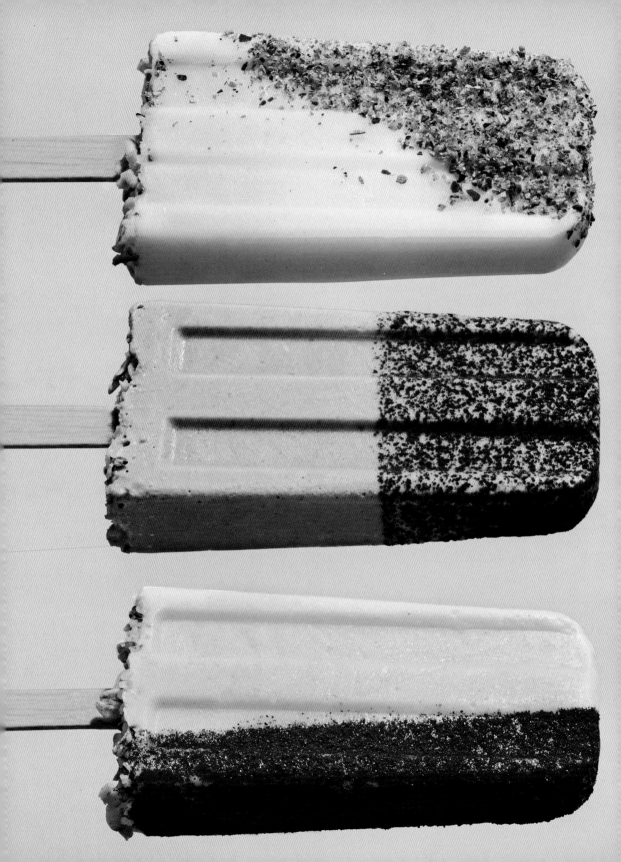

20 Creative Ways to Use
Greek Yogurt

If you're able to consume dairy, Greek yogurt should be a staple in your diet—and that's a fact.

→ **Totally delicious and packed with protein, the typical serving of Greek yogurt delivers around 16 grams of protein. But protein is not its only benefit! Greek yogurt also contains probiotics (that good-for-your-gut bacteria), plus a solid amount of both calcium and vitamin D. On top of all the health benefits, the amazing thing about Greek yogurt is that it's super versatile.**

You can use it in a wide range of recipes. It can be turned into a sauce, a delicious dessert, used as a substitute in cooking, or just eaten plain with toppings (which is great too!). Here's how to get the most out of your next tub.

1 ◀ Freeze It for Popsicles
Greek yogurt works well in popsicle form. Whitney Linsenmeryer, PhD, RD, LD, spokesperson for the Academy of Nutrition and Dietetics adds yogurt to a vegetable or fruit puree to make a delicious snack for later. "It gives a really nice creamy feeling and holds up well for different fruit flavors," she says.

2 Amp Up Your Overnight Oats
These just got way better. The breakfast dish is already packed with nutrients and fiber, so adding in some Greek yogurt makes it even healthier. One easy recipe includes oats, Greek yogurt, mashed banana, cinnamon, vanilla, and chia seeds. Combine the ingredients, let sit for at least two hours (or overnight), and enjoy.

3 Swap It as a Mayo Substitute
Greek yogurt makes a great substitute for any dish that calls for mayo. Add some canned tuna to Greek yogurt and you have a tasty dish at your fingertips. It only takes about 10 minutes.

4 Pump Up Your Smoothie
You can't go wrong by starting your day with a smoothie, and adding some Greek yogurt to your daily recipe can step it up. Plain pairs well with anything, but try adding in some peanut butter, too. For some easy recipes to boost with Greek yogurt turn to pages 42 to 47.

5 Whip Up Peanut Butter Dip

Greek yogurt peanut butter dip is a sweet, healthy dip to serve at your next gathering, says Linsenmeyer. All you need to do is mix the two ingredients together. "That can make a great dip for kids to eat with some fruits or veggies," she says.

6 Sub It for Cream in Pasta Sauce

If you're thinking about all those trips to Europe popping up on your feed, cure a bit of your FOMO by making some pasta sauce from scratch. Most creamy sauces call for half and half or heavy cream, which can easily be replaced with some Greek yogurt.

7 Replace Whipped Cream

This method is unconventional. You can swap out whipped cream, or any dish that's served à la mode, with some Greek yogurt. A scoop tastes so good on a warm fruit crisp, over banana splits, or on pancakes and waffles, and it's a nice way to balance out the sugar content of these foods with a hit of protein.

8 Give Soups a Boost

Similar to pasta sauce, Greek yogurt can make a great addition to creamy soups that call for heavy cream. If you prefer your soup meatless, this also adds a welcome dose of protein to the mix. Pro tip: Add it into your mixture last to keep it from separating.

9 Marinate Meats

Linsenmeyer also recommends using Greek yogurt as a marinade, particularly for chicken breast. "It marinates the protein much more slowly compared to a really strong acid," she says. "When it hits, it does really well on the grill."

10 Churn Homemade "Ice Cream"

This is a classic you've likely had before, even if you believed it was ice cream. Greek yogurt is delicious as a frozen treat with some berries or other fruit added on top (or mixed in.) To make, all you need is a food processor or blender, some fruit, and about 30 minutes (or more) to let the mixture chill in the freezer.

11 Create a Green Goddess Dressing

Dressing is another great opportunity for a Greek yogurt substitution. Linsenmeyer suggests using it to make green goddess dressing. She'll blend Greek yogurt with parsley, cilantro, and a little olive oil and vinegar. "Traditionally, a green goddess dressing is made with mayonnaise, so the yogurt is a nice substitute that gives it a ton of creaminess," she says.

12 Trade It for Baking Powder

Yup. You can bake a full-on cake with Greek yogurt. Yogurt has a high acidic pH, and it can also be mixed with baking soda to replace baking powder in any recipe that calls for it.

13 Decorate Baked Goods

A frosting that tastes good and has some protein? Count us in. You can mix Greek yogurt with some powdered sugar and make an excellent icing alternative. Just combine the ingredients and mix well.

14 Trade It for Sour Cream

This classic substitute cannot be overlooked! You may already know that plain Greek yogurt makes a much healthier alternative to sour cream, but it's worth a reminder. Add it to chili, tacos, quesadillas, or anything else that might call for some sour cream.

15 Dip Veggies in It

You can mix it with some dill and garlic powder and get an extremely tasty veggie dip, but plain old Greek yogurt also pairs well as a savory dip for some veggies. Try it with carrots or zucchini for an easy afternoon snack.

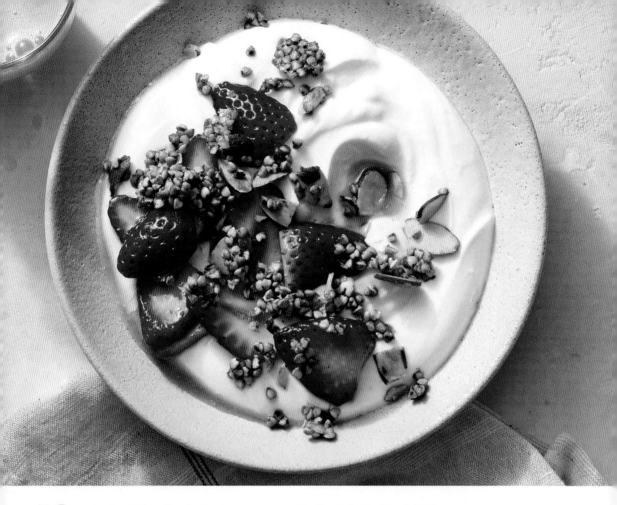

16 ⚠ **Layer It in a Parfait**
Greek yogurt is great on its own, but add in some fruit and granola to really level it up. A parfait makes a high-protein breakfast, or even a healthy dessert.

17 **Tone Down Spicy Dishes**
Any dish with lots of spice can be lightened up with some Greek yogurt. It helps with the creaminess too. Add your yogurt when it's at room temperature; otherwise, you might risk it separating.

18 **Add It to Your Charcuterie Board**
Sure, you've seen some spreadable cheeses and jams on charcuterie boards, but have you tried Greek yogurt? Its tart flavor will fit right in among your meats, breads, and nuts.

19 **Stir Up Tzatziki Sauce**
This authentic Greek recipe truly only takes 10 minutes, and it's so delicious: Grate some cucumbers, then mix together yogurt, some garlic, white vinegar, and a little olive oil. Then add the cucumbers to the mixture and let sit in the fridge for about 30 minutes. Boom! You have a delicious and surprisingly effortless tzatziki sauce.

20 **Make Cheese (Seriously!)**
Oh, yeah. This one is a little more complicated, but you can totally make cheese from Greek yogurt. Spoon some into a cheesecloth (or truly any clean cloth) and place in a strainer. Then place something heavy on top and leave it alone for a few days. This process will give you some spreadable, vegetarian-friendly cheese.

Lunches & Dinners

Choose from these satisfying, tasty, and **protein-packed** meals all day long.

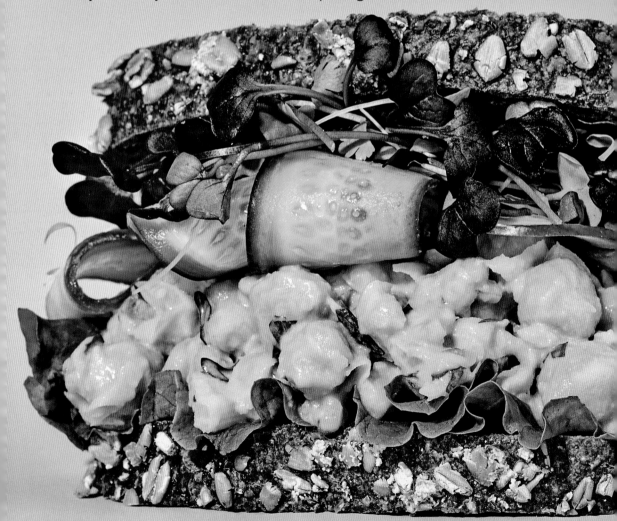

Chickpea Salad Sandwiches

TOTAL 10 MIN. **SERVES** 4

2	Tbsp fresh lemon juice
2	Tbsp vegan mayonnaise
1	Tbsp low-sodium soy sauce
1	Tbsp nutritional yeast
2	15-oz cans chickpeas, rinsed
2	stalks celery, thinly sliced
1	scallion, sliced
¼	cup cornichons (about 7), finely chopped
½	cup parsley, chopped
8	slices whole-grain bread
4	leaves green leaf lettuce
1	Persian cucumber or ½ seedless cucumber, peeled into ribbons
1	cup sprouts

1. In large bowl, whisk together lemon juice, mayonnaise, soy sauce, and nutritional yeast. Add chickpeas and mash, leaving some larger chunks. Fold in celery, scallion, cornichons, and parsley.

2. Assemble sandwiches with bread, lettuce, chickpea mixture, cucumber, and sprouts.

Per serving *About 472 calories, 12 g fat (2 g saturated fat), 2.5 mg cholesterol, 905 mg sodium, 70 g carbohydrates, 16 g fiber, 11.5 g sugars (0 g added sugars), 23 g protein*

POWER UP!
A study in the *Journal of Agricultural and Food Chemistry* found microgreens like sprouts can be up to 40 more potent in phytochemicals than mature varieties.

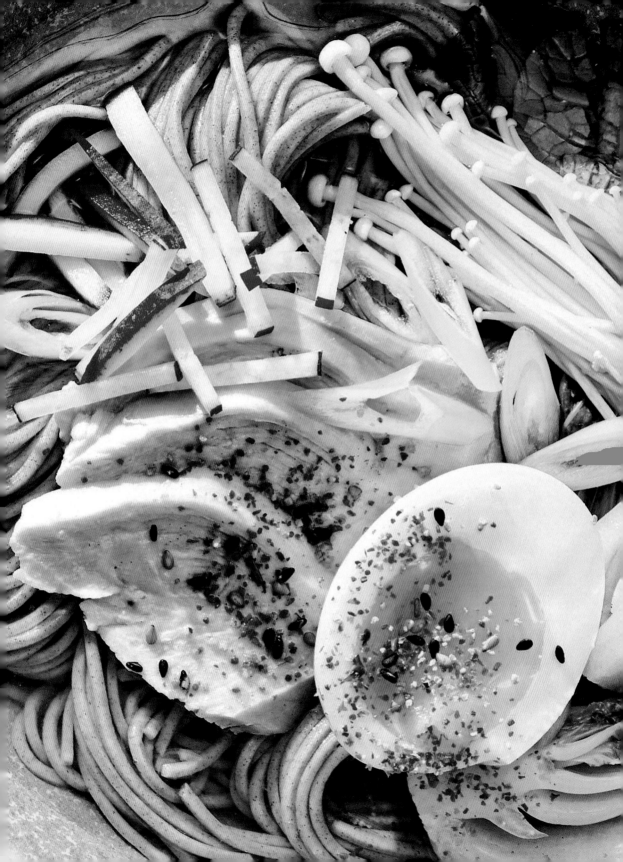

Bok Choy, Radish, and Chicken Soba in Dashi Broth

TOTAL 40 MIN. SERVES 4

8   scallions

2   6-in. pieces dried kombu (about 1 oz)

1   oz bonito flakes

6   oz soba noodles

4   cloves garlic, grated

1½   -in. piece ginger, peeled, thinly sliced, and then cut into matchsticks

2   Tbsp low-sodium tamari

2   heads baby bok choy, trimmed, leaves separated and halved lengthwise

12   oz boneless, skinless chicken breasts, very thinly sliced

2   Tbsp rice vinegar

2   cups tatsoi leaves

4   oz radishes (watermelon, purple, red, or daikon), cut into matchsticks

Soft-boiled eggs, enoki mushrooms, and togarashi, for serving

1. Halve scallions where they begin to turn green. Thinly slice greens and reserve; smash white parts. Put scallion whites in large saucepan along with kombu and 7 cups water. Bring to simmer on medium (about 10 min.). Once water begins to simmer, add bonito flakes, turn off heat, and steep 3 min. Strain liquid through a fine-mesh sieve into a clean pot.
2. Meanwhile, cook noodles per package directions.
3. Add garlic, ginger, and tamari to broth and bring to a boil. Stir in bok choy and turn off heat. Stir in chicken and half of scallion greens; let stand 1 min. Stir in vinegar and tatsoi.
4. Divide noodles and radishes among bowls and ladle soup on top. Serve topped with remaining scallions, eggs, mushrooms, and togarashi, if using.

Per serving *About 304 cal, 3 g fat (0.5 g sat fat), 174 mg chol, 493 mg sodium, 39 g carb, 5 g fiber, 3.5 g sugar (0 g added sugar), 29 g pro*

"
"Protein takes longer to digest and helps your body keep a steady supply of energy going into your bloodstream."

–Mary Ellen Phipps, MPH, RDN, author of The Easy Diabetes Cookbook.

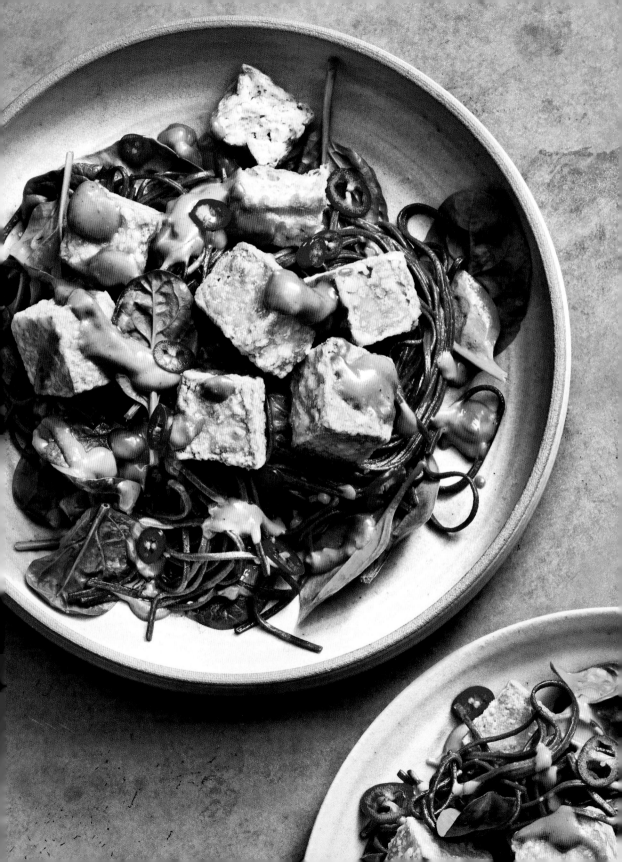

Air Fryer Tofu with Peanut Sauce and Soba

TOTAL 35 MIN. **SERVES** 4

2 12.3-oz packages extra-firm tofu, drained

3 Tbsp canola oil

2 tsp grated garlic, divided

2½ Tbsp low-sodium soy sauce, divided

3 Tbsp natural smooth peanut butter

1 Tbsp agave or honey

1 Tbsp fresh lime juice

¼ cup hot water

¼ tsp grated ginger

1 tsp sriracha

1 Tbsp toasted sesame oil

⅔ cup cornstarch

8 oz soba noodles, cooked per package directions

5 oz baby spinach

Sliced Fresno chiles, for serving

1. Pat tofu dry with paper towels and cut into ¾-inch cubes.

2. In small bowl, whisk together canola oil, half of garlic, and 1 Tbsp soy sauce. Transfer one-third to small baking dish, coating bottom evenly. Add tofu and pour remaining marinade on top. Gently turn tofu to coat and let sit at room temp 45 min.

3. In medium bowl, combine peanut butter, agave, and lime juice with remaining 1½ Tbsp soy sauce. Gradually whisk in hot water to emulsify. Whisk in ginger, sriracha, sesame oil, and remaining garlic. Set aside.

4. Heat air fryer to 400°F. Carefully dredge marinated tofu in cornstarch, coating evenly and shaking off excess. Add tofu to air fryer basket, spacing apart. Air-fry, shaking basket twice, until golden brown and crisp, 15 to 18 min.

5. Meanwhile, in large bowl, toss warm soba noodles with baby spinach and peanut sauce. Serve topped with crispy tofu and chiles, if using.

Per serving *About 697 calories, 29.5 g fat (3.5 g saturated fat), 0 mg cholesterol, 562 mg sodium, 79 g carbohydrates, 4 g fiber, 5.5 g sugar (4.5 g added sugar), 33 g protein*

Test Kitchen Trick **WHEN COOKING** soba noodles, do not salt the water. It can affect the texture and sturdiness of the noodles.

Thai-Style Peanut Chicken Wrap

TOTAL 25 MIN. **SERVES** 4

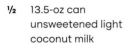

½ 13.5-oz can unsweetened light coconut milk

½ Tbsp plus ¼ tsp chili sauce

12 oz boneless, skinless chicken breasts, trimmed and cut into thin cutlets

4 large leaves Swiss chard

2 Tbsp crunchy peanut butter

1 tsp honey

½ tsp grated fresh ginger

2 Tbsp fresh lime juice, divided, plus lime wedges for serving

1 medium carrot (about 4 oz)

2 small Persian cucumbers

1 small red pepper, sliced

1. In large bowl, whisk together coconut milk and ½ Tbsp chili sauce. Reserve ½ cup mixture and set aside. Add chicken to remaining mixture and refrigerate at least 20 min. and up to 24 hr.
2. Meanwhile, fill large skillet with 1 inch water and bring to a simmer. Fill large bowl with ice water and line baking sheet with clean dish towels. Working with 1 chard leaf at a time, lay on work surface vein side up and carefully trim side of stem so it's level with rest of leaf (this will make it more pliable when wrapping). Add leaf to water and cook 30 seconds; transfer to ice water to cool, then transfer to baking sheet; repeat with remaining leaves.
3. Make peanut dipping sauce: In small bowl, whisk together peanut butter, honey, ginger, 1 Tbsp lime juice, 2 Tbsp reserved coconut mixture, and remaining ¼ tsp chili sauce; set aside.
4. Using vegetable peeler, cut carrot lengthwise into ribbons and toss with remaining 1 Tbsp lime juice; let sit, tossing occasionally, until ready to use.
5. Heat grill or grill pan on medium. Remove chicken from marinade (discard marinade) and grill until lightly charred on one side, 1 to 2 min. Flip and continue cooking, basting with some reserved coconut mixture, until chicken is cooked through, 3 to 6 min. more. Transfer chicken to cutting board, brush with any remaining coconut mixture, and let rest at least 5 min. before slicing.
6. Using vegetable peeler, cut cucumber into ribbons. Roll vegetables in chicken in a chard leaf, folding the sides over filling and rolling up from bottom. Serve with peanut sauce.

Per serving *About 207 calories, 8.5 g fat (3.5 g saturated), 47 mg cholesterol, 222mg sodium, 12g carbohydrates, 3g fiber, 6.5g sugar (1.5g added sugar), 21g protein*

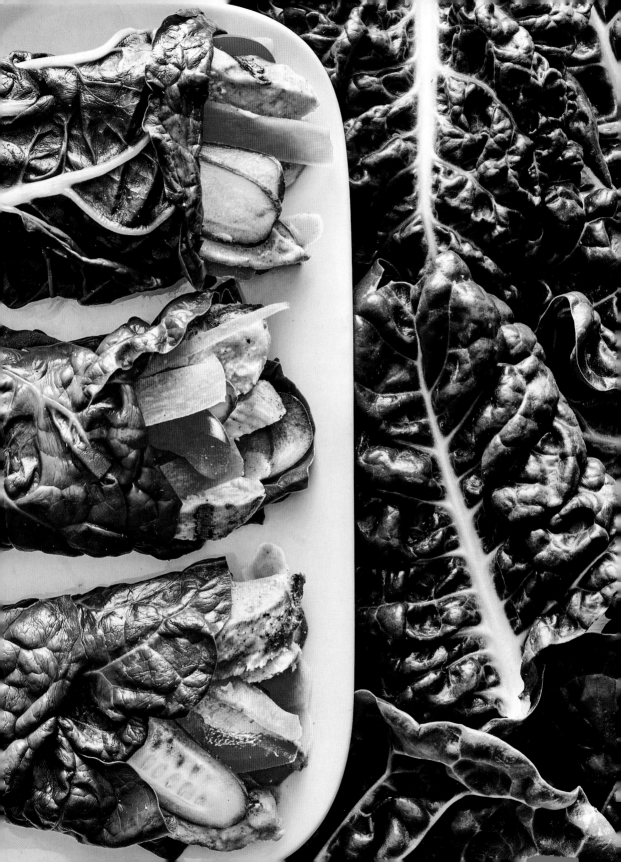

Chipotle Chicken Quinoa Soup

TOTAL 26 MIN. **SERVES** 1 TO 4

1½ Tbsp olive oil

1 onion, chopped

Kosher salt

½ medium butternut squash, about 12 oz, peeled and cut into ¾-inch pieces

1 medium poblano, cut into ¼-inch pieces

2 cloves garlic, pressed

1¼ tsp ground cumin

1 canned chipotle in adobo, finely chopped, plus 1 Tbsp adobo

3 cups bone or vegetable broth

2 6-oz boneless, skinless chicken breasts

1 14-oz can diced fire-roasted tomatoes

½ cup quinoa

1 15-oz can black beans, rinsed

⅓ cup cilantro, chopped, plus leaves for serving

⅓ cup roasted pepitas

1. Heat oil in Dutch oven on medium. Add onion and ½ tsp salt and cook, covered, stirring occasionally, for 6 min.
2. Add butternut squash and poblano and cook, stirring occasionally, for 4 min. Stir in garlic and cumin and cook 1 min.
3. Stir in chipotle and adobo, then broth. Add chicken and bring to a boil. When edges of pot just start bubbling, stir in tomatoes and quinoa, reduce heat, and simmer gently, covered, until chicken is cooked through and quinoa is tender, 12 to 14 min.
4. Transfer chicken to plate and when cool enough to handle, shred into pieces. Stir beans into soup and cook until heated through, about 3 min. Stir in chicken and cilantro and serve topped with pepitas and additional cilantro, if desired.

Per serving *About 488 calories, 14.5 g fat (2.5 g saturated fat), 3 mg cholesterol, 945 mg sodium, 50 g carbohydrates, 12 g fiber, 7.5 g sugar (0.5 g added sugar), 42 g protein*

POWER UP!
Bone broth adds about 10 grams of protein per serving. It's also a source of collagen and minerals and amino acids that benefit your gut, support joint health, and improve skin elasticity.

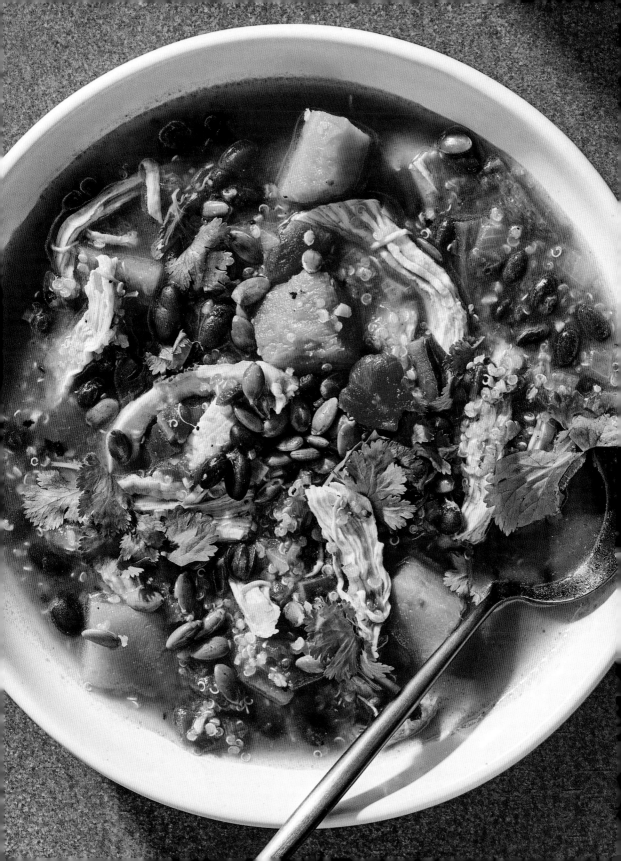

Chili with Wheat Berries and Beans

TOTAL 6 HR. 20 MIN. SERVES 4

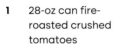

1	28-oz can fire-roasted crushed tomatoes
1	14.5-oz can low-salt diced tomatoes
1	Tbsp chili powder
2	tsp ground cumin
1	tsp ground coriander
3	cloves garlic, pressed
2	large poblano peppers, cut into ¼-inch pieces
1	onion, chopped
¾	cup wheat berries
	Kosher salt and pepper
½	bunch cilantro
2	15.5-oz cans low-sodium beans (one red kidney, one black), rinsed
½	sliced jalapeño, for serving
½	lime, for serving

1. In slow cooker, combine tomatoes (and their juices), chili powder, cumin, coriander, and ¾ cup water.

2. Stir in garlic, poblanos, onion, wheat berries, and ½ tsp each salt and pepper. Reserve 1 cup cilantro leaves, then tie the rest with kitchen twine and add to slow cooker. Cook, covered, until wheat berries are tender but still chewy, 5 to 6 hr. on High (or 7 to 8 hr. on Low).

3 Ten minutes before serving, gently stir in beans. Divide among bowls and top with reserved cilantro and jalapeño slices, if desired. Serve with lime wedges.

Per serving *About 423 calories, 1.5 g fat (0 g saturated fat), 0 mg cholesterol, 981 mg sodium, 83 g carbohydrates, 23 g fiber, 12.5 g sugar (0 g added sugar), 22.5 g protein*

POWER UP!
Wheat berries cook up with a firm, chewy texture and offer both protein and iron. Using them in slow-cooked recipes, like chili and stews, adds a hearty boost to the meal.

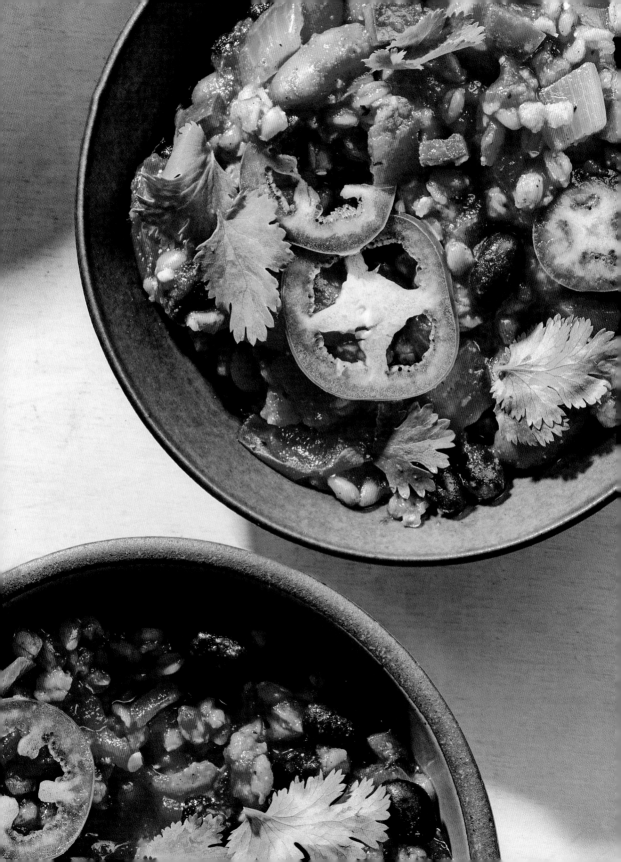

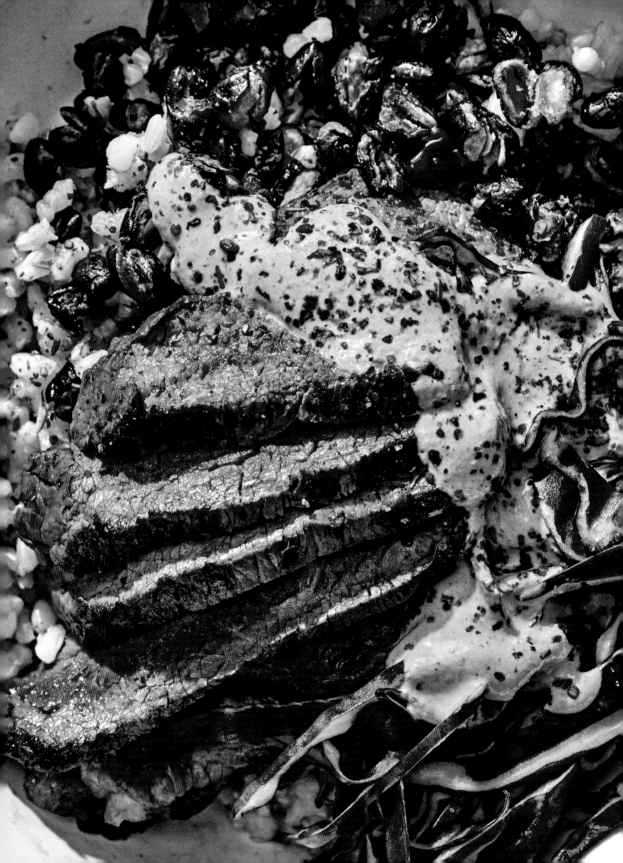

Steak Burrito Bowl Salad

TOTAL 30 MIN. **SERVES** 4

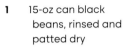

1   15-oz can black beans, rinsed and patted dry

3½ Tbsp olive oil, divided

1   tsp Tajín, plus more for sprinkling

1   1-lb sirloin steak (1½-inch thick), trimmed

Kosher salt and pepper

2   cups cilantro, chopped

1   small shallot, roughly chopped

½   jalapeño, seeded and roughly chopped

¼   cup fresh orange juice

2   Tbsp fresh lime juice

2   Tbsp Greek yogurt

2   cups cooked short-grain brown rice

¼   small head red cabbage (8 oz), cored and thinly sliced

1. Heat oven to 425°F. Add black beans to rimmed baking sheet and toss with ½ Tbsp oil and Tajín. Roast until beans are dry, split, and crispy, 18 to 20 min.

2. Meanwhile, heat 1 Tbsp oil in large cast-iron skillet on medium-high. Pat steak completely dry and season with ½ tsp each salt and pepper. Cook to desired doneness, 5 to 6 min. per side for medium-rare. Transfer to cutting board and let rest at least 5 min. before slicing.

3. Meanwhile, in blender, combine cilantro, shallot, jalapeño, orange and lime juices, yogurt, and remaining 2 Tbsp oil. Puree on high until homogeneous but still bright green, 30 seconds.

4. Divide rice among bowls. Top with cabbage and roasted black beans. Add sliced steak and drizzle with green sauce and sprinkle with more Tajín, if desired.

Per serving About 570 calories, 28.5 g fat (8 g saturated fat), 76 mg cholesterol, 726 mg sodium, 48 g carbohydrates, 9 g fiber, 5 g sugar (0 g added sugar), 32 g protein

Test Kitchen Trick IF YOU don't have steak on hand prepare this dish with lean ground beef, grilled chicken, tofu, or your favorite plant-based protein.

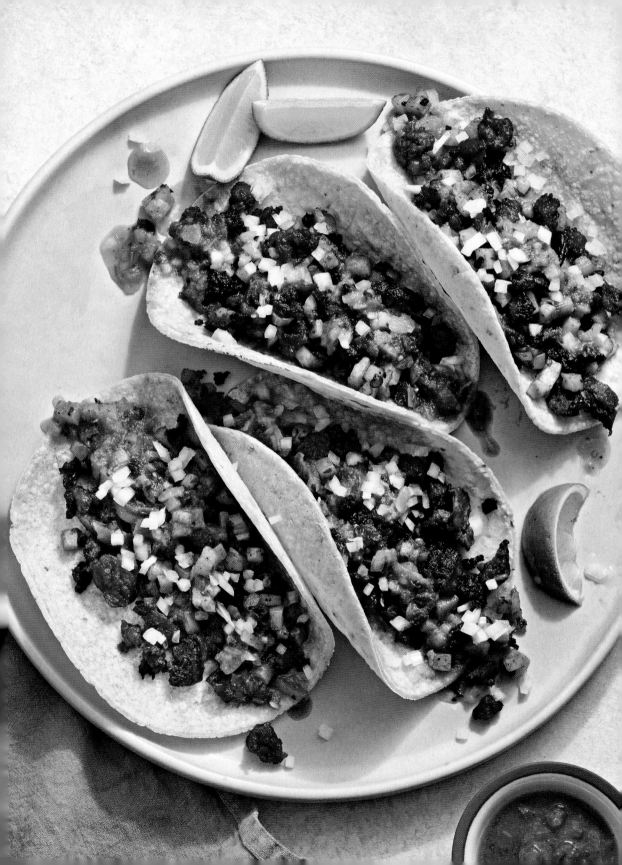

Chorizo and Potato Tacos

TOTAL 35 MIN. **SERVES** 4

1 Tbsp olive oil

1 lb fresh Mexican chorizo, casings discarded, crumbled into small pieces

1¼ lb russet potatoes (2 medium), cut into ¼-inch pieces

½ large white onion, finely chopped, divided

Salt

Ground black pepper

8 small corn tortillas, warmed

½ cup salsa verde, for serving

1. Heat 1 Tbsp olive oil in large cast-iron skillet on medium-high. Add chorizo and cook, undisturbed, until browned on bottom, 3 min. Continue to cook, breaking up into very small pieces and adjusting heat if burning, until very crisp and brown, 6 to 8 min. more. Using slotted spoon, transfer to bowl and pour off all but 1 Tbsp fat.

2. While chorizo cooks, in large bowl, microwave potatoes, covered with damp paper towel, until tender, 4 to 5 min.

3. Add cooked potatoes to skillet, arrange in single layer, and cook, stirring every few minutes, until golden brown, 5 to 7 min. Add all but ⅓ cup onion and ½ tsp each salt and pepper and cook, tossing every minute or so, until tender, 3 to 5 min.

4. Return chorizo to skillet and toss to combine. Spoon chorizo-potato mixture into tortillas; top with salsa verde and remaining ⅓ cup white onion.

Per serving *About 542 calories, 24 g fat (10 g saturated fat), 81 mg cholesterol, 1,203 mg sodium, 49 g carbohydrates, 5 g fiber, 7 g sugar (0 g added sugar), 25 g protein*

POWER UP!
Potatoes in the taco fillings add protein—yes really. For other high-protein veggies, turn to page 149.

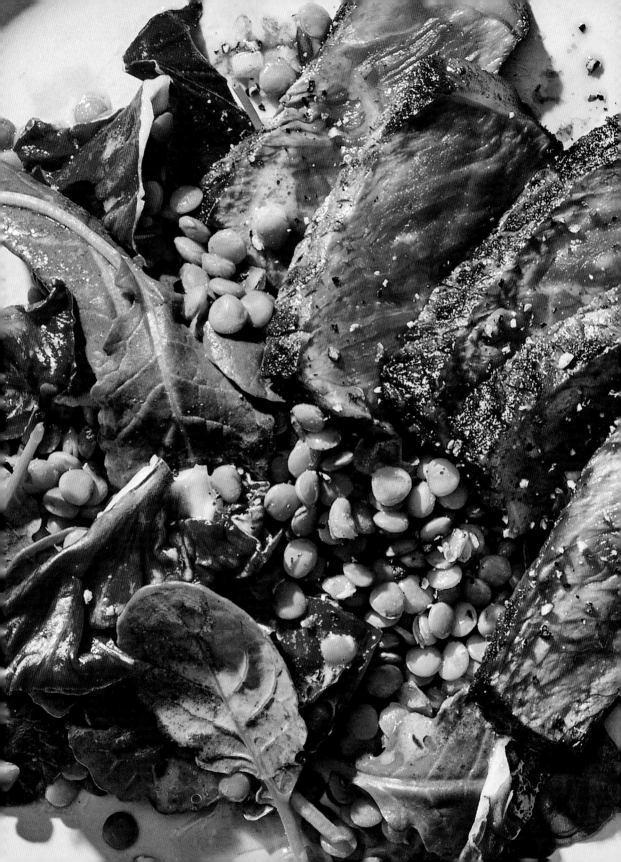

Smoky Steak and Lentil Salad

TOTAL 30 MIN. **SERVES** 4

1 Tbsp lemon juice

1 tsp Dijon mustard

Kosher salt and pepper

½ small red onion, finely chopped

2 1-inch-thick strip steaks (1½ lbs total), trimmed

1 Tbsp smoked paprika, plus more for serving

2 Tbsp olive oil, divided

1 15-oz can lentils, rinsed

½ head radicchio, chopped

2 cups baby kale

1. In large bowl, whisk together lemon juice, mustard, and ¼ tsp each salt and pepper; stir in onion and let sit 5 min.

2. Meanwhile, pat steaks dry with paper towels, then rub with paprika and ½ tsp each salt and pepper; shake off any excess.

3. Heat 1 Tbsp oil in large skillet on medium. Add steak and cook to desired doneness, 4 to 5 min. per side for medium-rare. Transfer to cutting board and let rest at least 5 min. before slicing.

4. Add lentils to onion and toss to combine. Toss with radicchio, kale, remaining Tbsp oil, and ¼ tsp each salt and pepper. Serve with sliced steak.

Per serving *About 498 calories, 26.5 g fat (9 g saturated fat), 94 mg cholesterol, 680 mg sodium, 18 g carbohydrates, 9 g fiber, 2.5 g sugars (0 g added sugars), 45 g protein*

FIBER FIX

Lentils are high in soluble fiber and one cup of cooked lentils contains 16 grams of fiber. They are also a great source of folate, a B vitamin, magnesium, and iron.

Pork, Pineapple, and Onion Skewers

TOTAL 45 MIN. **SERVES** 4

1 lb pork loin, trimmed and cut into 1-inch pieces

½ small pineapple (about 1 lb), trimmed, cored, and cut into 1-in. pieces (about 2 cups)

1 small red onion, cut into 6 wedges, each halved crosswise

8 oz baby peppers (mixed colors), cut into 1-inch pieces

2 Tbsp olive oil

Kosher salt and pepper

Teriyaki sauce, for basting

1 sliced jalapeño, for serving

1. In large bowl, toss pork, pineapple, onion, and peppers with oil and ½ tsp each salt and pepper.

2. Thread pork and vegetables onto skewers. Grill, turning occasionally, until pork is cooked through, 8 to 10 min. total, basting with teriyaki sauce during last 5 min. of cooking. Top with sliced jalapeño.

Per serving About 310 calories, 11 g fat (2.5 g saturated fat), 95 mg cholesterol, 895 mg sodium, 24 g carbohydrates, 2 g fiber, 16 g sugar (0 g added sugar), 29 g protein

Test Kitchen Trick **WOODEN SKEWERS**, like bamboo, **can burn easily on the grill. To prevent this, soak them in warm water for 10 to 30 minutes before threading food onto them.**

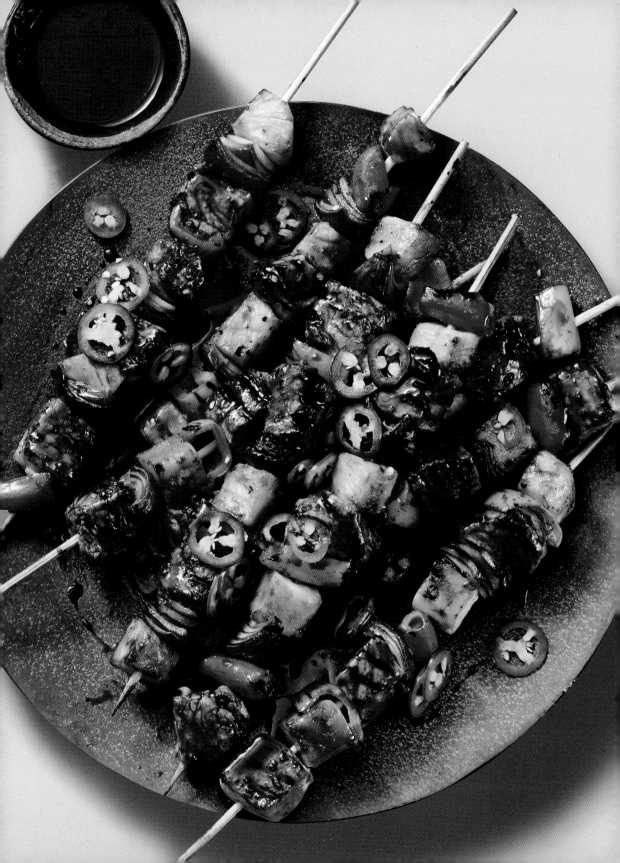

Fennel-Rubbed Pork Tenderloin with Broccoli Rabe and Roman Beans

TOTAL 30 MIN. **SERVES** 4

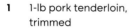

1   1-lb pork tenderloin, trimmed

3   Tbsp plus ½ tsp olive oil, divided

Kosher salt

1   Tbsp fennel seeds, crushed

1   16-oz bunch broccoli rabe, tough ends discarded, cut into bite-size pieces

4   large cloves garlic, finely chopped, divided

1   oz pecorino romano cheese

1   5.5-oz can roman beans, drained and liquid reserved

¼   tsp red pepper flakes

1   tsp lemon zest plus 2 Tbsp lemon juice

1. Heat oven to 450°F. Coat pork with ½ tsp oil, season with ¼ tsp salt, and rub with fennel seeds. Heat 1 Tbsp oil in large ovenproof skillet on medium-high. Add pork and cook, reducing heat to medium as needed to avoid burning, until deep golden brown on all sides, 6 to 7 min. total.

2. Transfer skillet to oven and roast until pork registers 145°F on instant-read thermometer, 4 to 6 min.

3. Meanwhile, on rimmed baking sheet, toss broccoli rabe with 2 Tbsp oil and ¼ tsp salt. Roast 5 min. then toss half of garlic into broccoli rabe. Continue roasting until tender and beginning to crisp around edges, 2 min. more. Grate pecorino romano on top.

4. Transfer pork to cutting board and let rest at least 5 min. before slicing (reserve skillet).

5. Add remaining garlic to reserved skillet and cook on medium, stirring, 30 sec. Stir in beans, ¼ cup reserved bean liquid, and red pepper flakes and cook until heated through, about 2 min. Stir in lemon juice.

6. Serve broccoli rabe topped with beans and pork and drizzled with any pan juices, then sprinkle with lemon zest.

Per serving *About 382 calories, 17.5 g fat (4 g saturated fat), 81 mg cholesterol, 773 mg sodium, 22 g carbohydrates, 10 g fiber, 0.5 g sugar (0 g added sugar), 35 g protien*

Prep Ahead   **WHILE PREPARING** the recipe above, double up and prepare twice the pork. Wrap and refrigerate for up to 3 days. Slice and pile on sandwiches or chop and toss into salads and grain bowls.

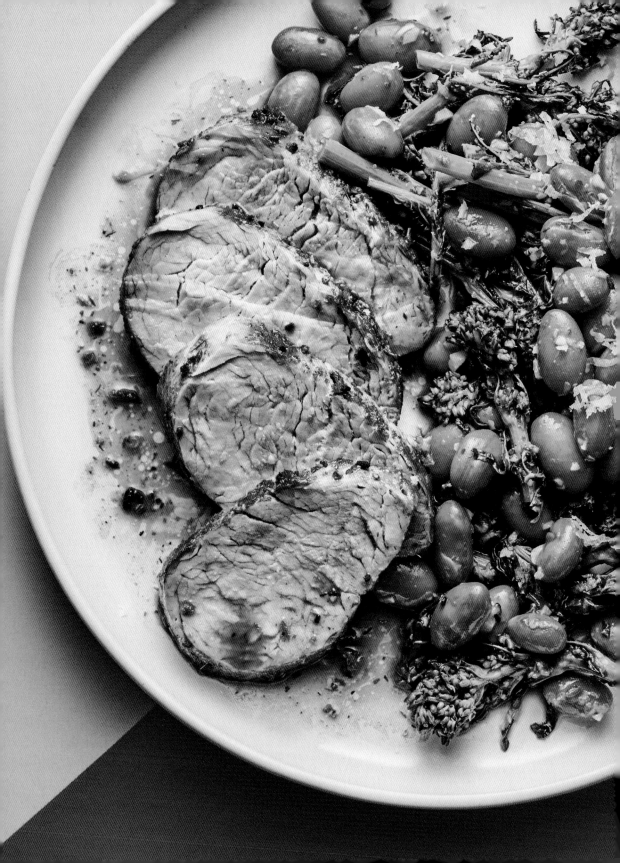

Sausage and Fennel Chickpea Rigatoni

TOTAL 25 MIN. **SERVES** 4

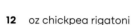

12 oz chickpea rigatoni

3 Tbsp olive oil, divided

1 Tbsp fennel seeds, crushed

1 lb Italian turkey sausage, casings removed

¼ cup low-sodium chicken broth or water

1 large bulb fennel, cored and thinly sliced

Kosher salt

2 cloves garlic, finely chopped

½ tsp red pepper flakes

2 tsp fresh lemon juice

¼ cup plus 2 Tbsp grated pecorino romano

6 cups baby kale

1. Cook pasta per package directions, stirring occasionally to prevent sticking. Reserve 1 cup cooking water; drain and rinse pasta.

2. Meanwhile, heat 2 Tbsp oil in large skillet on medium. Quickly add fennel seeds and bite-size pieces of sausage on top, gently pressing with spatula. Cook on medium-high, undisturbed, until golden brown on bottom, 4 to 6 min. Toss and cook just until cooked through, 1 to 2 min.; transfer to bowl. Add chicken broth (or water) to same skillet and bring to a simmer, scraping bottom of pan. Transfer to bowl with sausage.

3. Wipe out skillet and heat remaining Tbsp oil on medium. Add sliced fennel and ½ tsp salt and cook, stirring occasionally, until just tender, about 4 min. Stir in garlic and red pepper flakes and cook 1 min. Stir in lemon juice and ½ cup reserved cooking liquid.

4. Gently fold pasta and ¼ cup cheese into sliced fennel, then kale and half of sausage, adding more cooking liquid if pasta seems dry. Serve topped with remaining sausage and 2 Tbsp pecorino romano.

Per serving *About 638 calories, 30.5 g fat (6.5 g saturated fat), 77 mg cholesterol, 1,062 mg sodium, 56 g carbohydrates, 16 g fiber, 10.5 g sugar (0 g added sugar), 46 g protein*

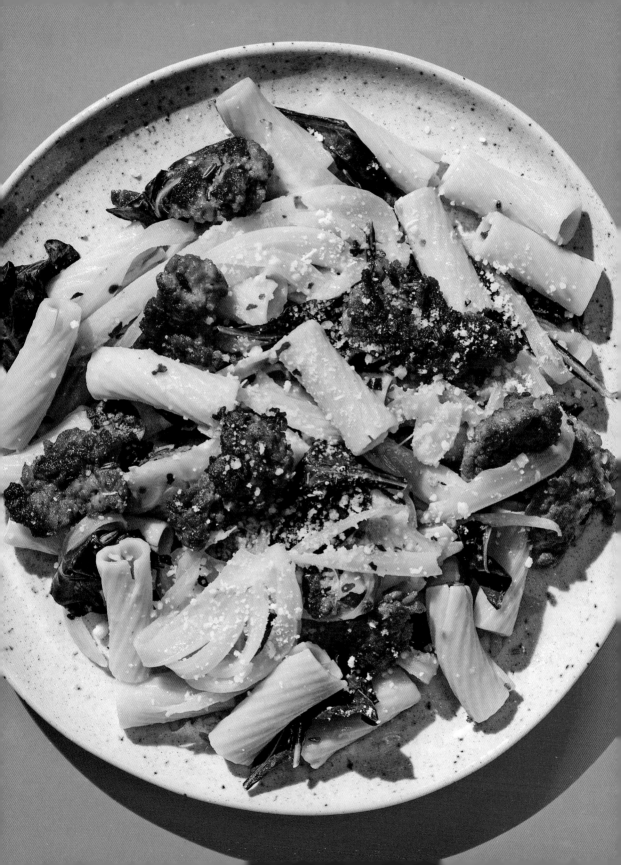

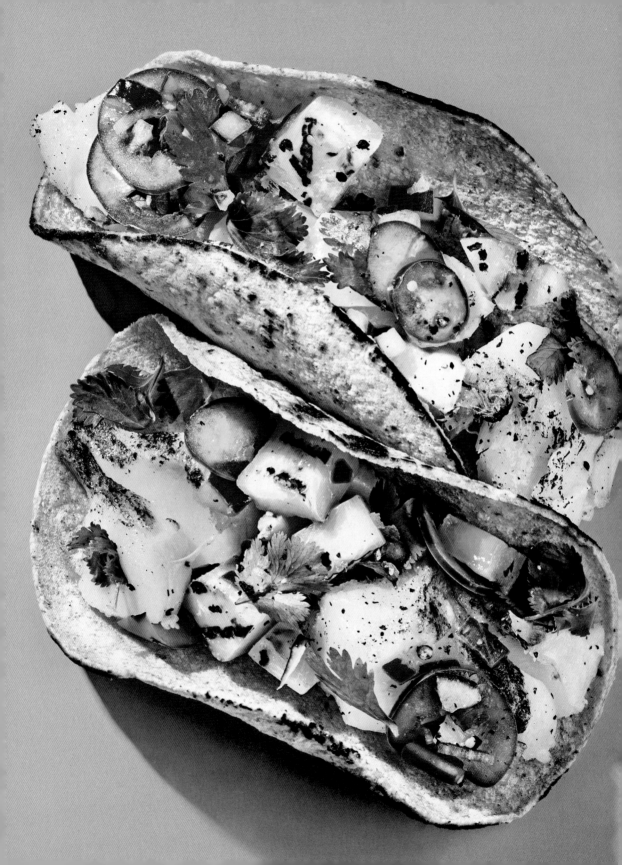

Grilled Fish Tacos with Charred Pineapple

TOTAL 20 MIN. **SERVES** 4

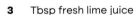

3 Tbsp fresh lime juice

½ small red onion, finely chopped

1 jalapeño, thinly sliced

Kosher salt and pepper

¼ small pineapple, sliced into thick rings

1¼ lbs skinless white fish fillets (such as tilapia, cod, or halibut)

1 Tbsp olive oil

¾ cup fresh cilantro leaves

8 corn tortillas, lightly charred

1. In a bowl, combine lime juice, onion, jalapeño, and ¼ tsp each salt and pepper.

2. Heat grill to medium-high. Grill pineapple until charred and beginning to soften, 2 to 3 min. per side.

3. Brush fish with oil, season with ¼ tsp each salt and pepper, and grill until lightly charred and opaque throughout, 2 to 5 min. per side (depending on the fish).

4. Cut pineapple into ½-inch pieces and toss with red onion mixture; fold in cilantro. Fill tortillas with fish and top with salsa.

Per serving About 234 calories, 5.5 g fat (0.5 g saturated fat), 0 mg cholesterol, 324 mg sodium, 23 g carbohydrates, 2 g fiber, 7 g sugars (0 g added sugars), 25 g protein

Test Kitchen Trick **TO CRISP** your tortillas over a gas flame, adjust the heat to medium low. Using tongs, place the tortilla directly over the flame. Warm tortilla until charred, about 15 to 30 seconds, and then flip to cook the other side.

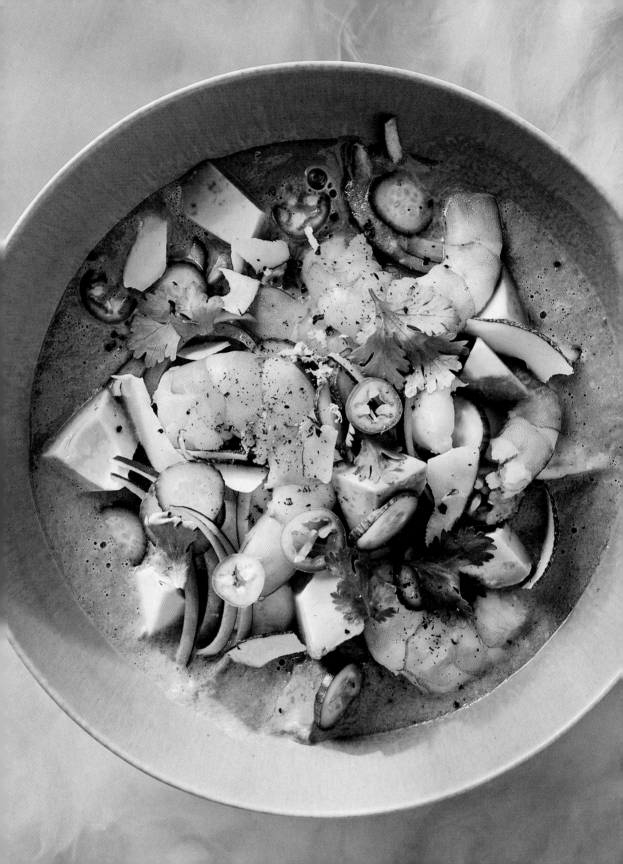

Shrimp, Cucumber, and Tomatillo Chilled Soup

TOTAL 1 HR. 25 MIN. **SERVES** 4

- **3** medium serrano chiles (stemmed and seeded for less heat, if desired), plus more sliced, for serving
- **1** large tomatillo (about 4 oz), peeled, rinsed, and cored
- **1** large clove garlic
- **5** Tbsp fresh lime juice
- **1¼** cup bottled coconut water (from refrigerator section)
- **1½** cup cilantro, plus extra leaves, for serving
- **1½** Tbsp canola oil
- **3** Persian cucumbers, half chopped into large chunks and half thinly sliced

Kosher salt

- **1** lb extra-large cooked, peeled, and deveined shrimp (thawed, if frozen), halved horizontally
- **½** small red onion, thinly sliced
- **1½** oz fresh coconut, shaved
- **1** avocado, diced

1. In blender on high, purée serranos, tomatillo, garlic, lime juice, coconut water, cilantro, oil, chopped cucumber, and 1 tsp salt until smooth, about 30 seconds. Refrigerate in airtight container until completely chilled, at least 1 hr., up to 3 days.

2. When ready to serve, toss shrimp with onion, sliced cucumber, and half of coconut. Pile mixture in serving bowls, then ladle in aguachile. Top with avocado, remaining coconut, sliced serrano, and cilantro leaves, if desired.

Per serving About 343 calories, 18.5 g fat (5.5 g saturated fat), 239 mg cholesterol, 1,581 mg sodium, 18 g carbohydrates, 6 g fiber, 7 g sugar (2 g added sugar), 28 g protein

FIBER FIX
Soups, especially cold soups, preserve the fiber in produce. They also offer protein, fat, and seasonings which help with satiety.

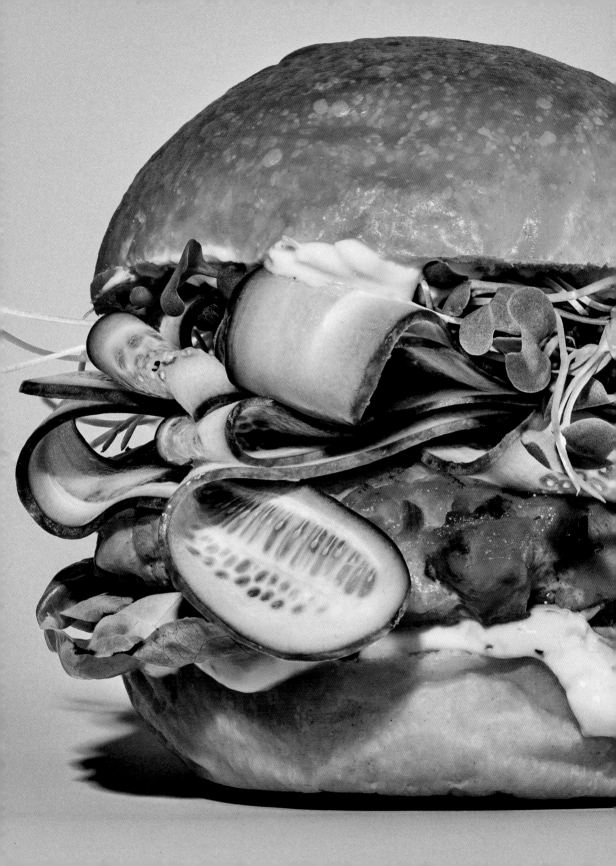

Salmon Burgers

TOTAL 30 MIN. **SERVES** 4

1	large egg
1	lb skinless salmon fillet, finely chopped
2	scallions, chopped
1	jalapeño, finely chopped
3	Tbsp cilantro, chopped, divided
	Kosher salt and pepper
1	Tbsp olive oil
½	cup Greek yogurt
1	tsp lime zest plus 2 Tbsp juice
4	brioche buns, toasted
8	Bibb lettuce leaves
2	Persian cucumbers or ½ English cucumber, shaved lengthwise
2	cups broccoli or radish sprouts

1. In medium bowl, beat egg until frothy. Fold in salmon, scallions, jalapeño, 2 Tbsp cilantro, ½ tsp salt, and ¼ tsp pepper.

2. Heat oil in large nonstick skillet on medium. Spoon 4 mounds of salmon mixture (about ½ cup each) into skillet and flatten into ½-in. thick patties. Cook until golden brown, 2 min. per side.

3. Meanwhile, in bowl, combine yogurt, lime zest and juice, remaining Tbsp cilantro, and ¼ tsp each salt and pepper and spread on buns. Top bottom buns with lettuce, salmon patties, cucumber, and sprouts; sandwich with top buns.

Per serving *About 379 calories, 13 g fat (3.5 g saturated fat), 134 g cholesterol, 580 mg sodium, 32 g carbohydrates, 8.5 g sugars (0 g added sugars), 3 g fiber, 34 g protein*

POWER UP!
Research from the journal *Future of Oncology* found that sulforaphane, a compound found in broccoli microgreens, has the potential to target cancer stem cells.

Sheet Pan Salmon and Tomatoes

TOTAL 30 MIN. **SERVES** 4

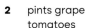

2 pints grape tomatoes

2 Tbsp olive oil

1½ tsp coriander seeds, crushed

½ tsp cumin seeds, crushed

Kosher salt and pepper

1 lb skinless salmon fillet, cut into 1½-in. pieces

2 scallions, thinly sliced, divided

2 cups baby kale

Greek yogurt and crumbled feta, for serving

4 small pieces flatbread, naan, or pita, warmed, for serving

1. Heat oven to 450°F. On rimmed baking sheet, toss tomatoes, oil, coriander, cumin, and ¼ tsp each salt and pepper. Roast 12 min.

2. Season salmon with ¼ tsp each salt and pepper and nestle among tomatoes. Reduce oven temp to 425°F and continue roasting until tomatoes have begun to break down and are juicy, and salmon is opaque throughout, 8 to 10 min. more.

3. Scatter half of scallions, then kale, over salmon and tomatoes; let sit 2 min.

4. Spread yogurt on flatbreads, top with salmon and vegetables, then sprinkle with feta and remaining scallion, if desired.

Per serving *About 595 calories, 21 g fat (4.5 g saturated fat), 63 mg cholesterol, 1,100 mg sodium, 68.5 g carbohydrates, 4 g fiber, 5 g sugar (0 g added sugar), 36 g protein*

POWER UP!
Salmon is a buttery fish that's rich in omega-3 fatty acids and protein and a solid source of bone-building calcum and energy-revving iron.

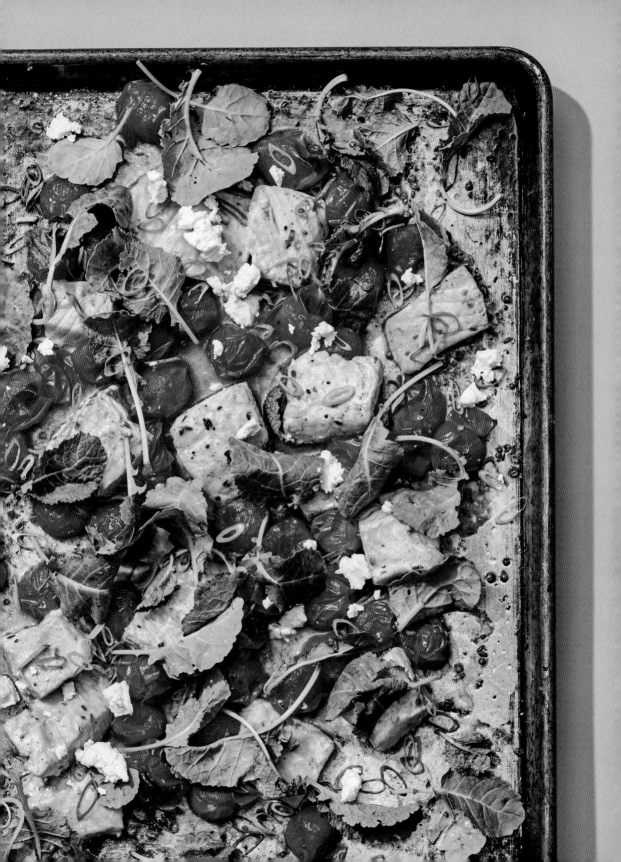

Halibut With Citrus Endive Salad

TOTAL 10 MIN. **SERVES** 4

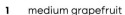

1	medium grapefruit
1	Cara cara orange
3	Tbsp white wine vinegar
2½	Tbsp olive oil, divided
½	tsp honey

Kosher salt and pepper

2	medium shallots, finely chopped
4	5-oz skinless fillets halibut
3	small heads endive (combo of red and green), leaves separated
1	head fennel, cored and very thinly sliced
⅓	cup mint leaves, roughly chopped, plus whole mint leaves for serving
1	small avocado, sliced
¼	cup shelled, roasted pistachios, chopped (optional)

1. Grate 2 tsp zest from grapefruit into large bowl. Cut tops and bottoms off grapefruit and orange, cut peel and pith away, then cut segments from between membranes and transfer to plate. Squeeze 1½ Tbsp juice from remaining membranes into bowl with zest; add vinegar, 1½ Tbsp oil, honey, and ½ tsp each salt and pepper and whisk to combine; stir in shallots and let sit 5 min.

2. Meanwhile, heat remaining 1 Tbsp oil in large nonstick skillet on medium. Season fish with ¼ tsp each salt and pepper and cook, undisturbed, until golden brown on bottom, about 3 min. Flip and cook until opaque, about 2 min. more.

3 Add endive, fennel, and mint to shallot mixture and toss to combine. Gently fold in grapefruit and orange segments along with avocado. Serve with fish, topped with pistachios and additional mint leaves, if desired.

Per serving About 454 calories, 20.5 g fat (3 g saturated fat), 77 mg cholesterol, 566 mg sodium, 36 g carbohydrates, 17 g fiber, 15 g sugar (0.5 g added sugar), 37 g protein

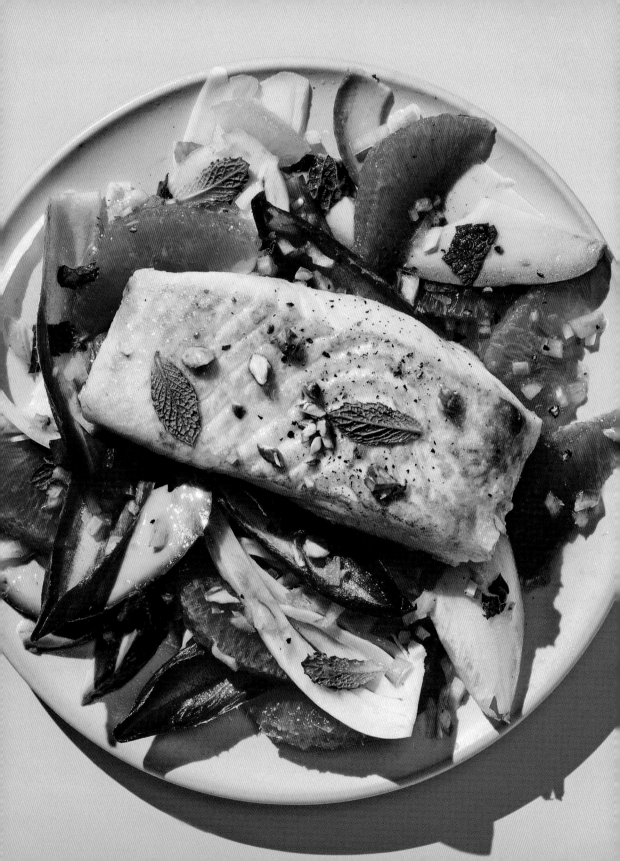

Gochujang Shrimp and Cabbage Stew

TOTAL 35 MIN. **SERVES** 4

1	cup forbidden (black) rice or medium grain rice
3	Tbsp gochujang
1	Tbsp avocado oil or other neutral oil
1	red pepper, cut into 1-in. chunks
6	scallions, cut into 2-in. pieces, pale pieces halved lengthwise
3	cloves garlic, finely chopped
1	small head or ½ large head napa cabbage (about 12 oz), leaves cut into 2-in. pieces
1	bunch broccolini, long stems thinly sliced and tops cut into large florets
1	lb large peeled and deveined shrimp
⅓	cup basil, roughly chopped

1. Cook rice per package directions.
2. Meanwhile, in bowl, whisk together gochujang and 2 cups warm water to dissolve.
3. Heat oil in large, straight-sided saucepan on medium. Add pepper and cook, tossing for 3 min.
4. Increase heat to high and add scallions and garlic and cook, stirring, 1 min. Add cabbage and cook, tossing, 1 min. Stir in gochujang broth and bring to a steady simmer.
5. Layer broccolini on top of cabbage mixture, then scatter shrimp on top of that. Cover and cook 2 min. Flip shrimp and simmer, covered, until shrimp are opaque throughout and broccolini is just tender, 1 to 2 min. more. Stir in basil and serve over rice

PER SERVING: *About 361 calories, 6.5 g fat (0.5 g saturated fat), 143 mg cholesterol, 1,524 mg sodium, 56 g carbohydrates, 7 g fiber, 10.5 g sugar (0 g added sugar), 24 g protein*

FIBER FIX
Forbidden (black) rice is rich with antioxidants and fiber. This deep purple grain delivers 2 grams fiber and 5 grams protein per ½ cup prepared rice.

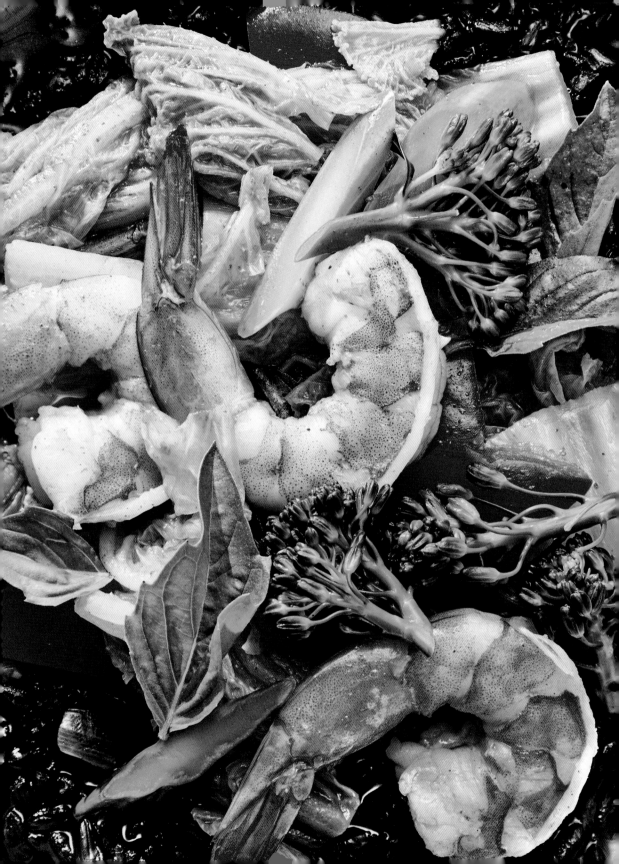

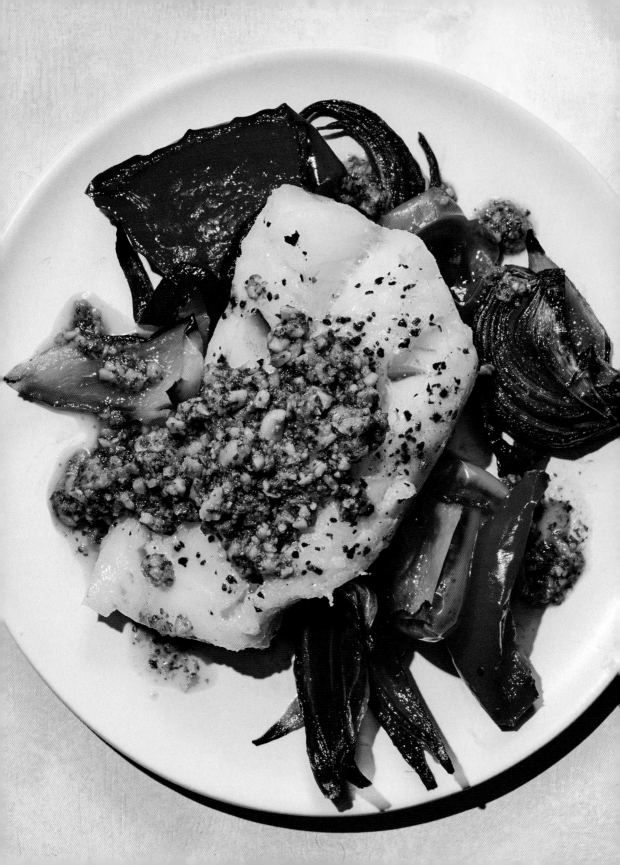

Roasted Fish and Peppers with Chickpea Pesto

TOTAL 45 MIN. **SERVES** 4

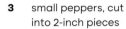

3   small peppers, cut into 2-inch pieces

1   medium red onion, cut into ½-inch-thick wedges

½   cup plus 1 Tbsp olive oil, divided

Kosher salt and pepper

4   6-oz firm white fish fillets (like cod)

½   tsp Aleppo pepper

Basil leaves

1½   Tbsp grated lemon zest plus 3 Tbsp juice (from 1 large lemon)

2   small cloves garlic

1   15-oz can low-sodium chickpeas, rinsed

1. Heat oven to 425°F. On rimmed baking sheet, toss peppers and onion with 1 Tbsp oil and ¼ tsp each salt and pepper. Roast until tender and beginning to brown, 20 to 22 min.

2. Season fish with Aleppo pepper and ½ tsp salt; nestle amid vegetables and roast until vegetables are golden brown and tender and fish is opaque throughout, 10 to 12 min. more.

3. Meanwhile, in food processor, pulse basil, lemon zest and juice, garlic, and ¼ tsp salt until finely chopped. Add remaining ½ cup oil and process until smooth. Add chickpeas and pulse until chopped but still slightly chunky. Serve pesto with fish and vegetables.

Per serving About 521 calories, 33.5 g fat (4.5 g saturated fat), 65 mg cholesterol, 646 mg sodium, 23 g carbohydrates, 6 g fiber, 5.5 g sugar (0 g added sugar), 34 g protein

POWER UP!
Protein in fish plays an essential role in neurotransmitter function, which supports good cognitive and mental health.

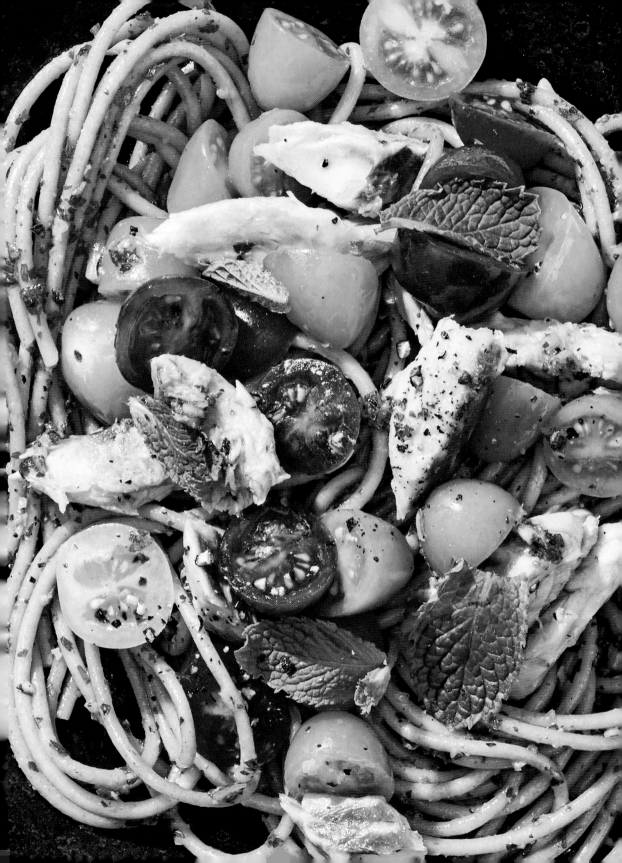

Mackerel and Tomato Pasta with Almond Mint Pesto

TOTAL 30 MIN. **SERVES** 4

10 oz whole-wheat spaghetti

3 4.4-oz cans boneless mackerel fillets in olive oil

12 oz mixed-color cherry tomatoes, halved (or quartered if large)

Kosher salt and pepper

2 cup mint leaves, plus more for serving

1 cup flat-leaf parsley leaves

1 large shallot, roughly chopped

4 fillets oil-packed anchovies, coarsely chopped

½ cup olive oil

⅔ cup roasted sliced almonds, divided

1. Cook pasta per package directions; drain and rinse under cold water to cool.

2. Meanwhile, drain mackerel, reserving 2 Tbsp oil; transfer mackerel to medium bowl and break into bite-size pieces. Gently toss with tomatoes, reserved mackerel oil, and a pinch each of salt and pepper.

3. In food processor, pulse mint, parsley, shallot, anchovies, and ¼ tsp each salt and pepper to finely chop. Add olive oil and ⅓ cup almonds and pulse until nuts are finely chopped.

4. In large bowl, toss pasta with almond mint pesto. Spoon mackerel salad on top and scatter with remaining almonds and additional mint leaves, if desired.

Per serving *About 884 calories, 54.4 g fat (7.5 g saturated fat), 33 mg cholesterol, 541 mg sodium, 74 g carbohydrates, 15 g fiber, 4 g sugar (0 g added sugar), 33 g protein*

Test Kitchen Trick TINNED FISH is a pantry staple and a protein powerhouse for weeknight meals. Flip to page 144 to read more about this convenient pantry staple.

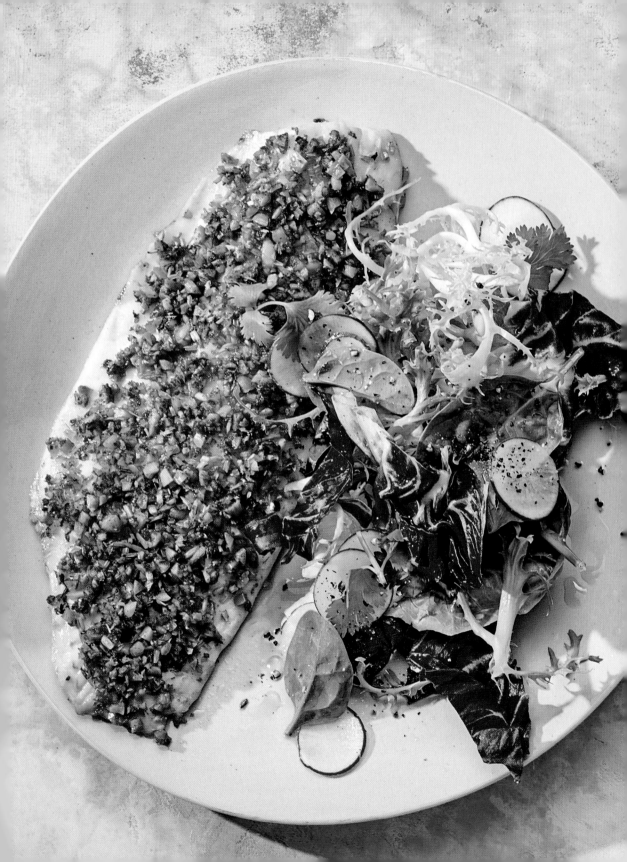

Almond-Crusted Striped Bass

TOTAL 35 MIN. **SERVES** 4

2 Tbsp extra-virgin olive oil, divided

4 5 oz boneless, skinless striped bass fillets

¼ bunch fresh cilantro

⅔ cup blanched, slivered almonds, toasted and roughly chopped

1 medium shallot, finely chopped (⅓ cup)

2 tsp grated lime zest plus 1 Tbsp juice, plus wedges for serving

1¼ tsp smoked paprika

1 tsp ground cumin

½ tsp ground cinnamon

¼ tsp ground allspice

Kosher salt and pepper

6 cups mixed greens

4 small radishes, thinly sliced

1. Heat oven to 375°F. Line rimmed baking sheet with parchment paper and brush with 1 tsp olive oil. Pat fillets dry with paper towels and lay on parchment.

2. From cilantro, finely chop stems to equal ⅓ cup and set aside ½ cup leaves for salad. In medium bowl, toss together cilantro stems, almonds, shallots, lime zest, smoked paprika, cumin, cinnamon, allspice, ½ tsp salt, and 2 tsp oil. Season fish with ¼ tsp each salt and pepper and divide almond mixture among fillets, spreading it to coat surface of fish and pressing to adhere. Roast until fish is just opaque throughout, 10 to 14 min.

3. Meanwhile, in large bowl, combine lime juice with remaining Tbsp oil. Add greens, radishes, reserved cilantro leaves, and pinch each of salt and pepper and toss to coat. Serve with lime wedges, if desired.

Per serving *About 340 calories, 20 g fat (2.5 g saturated fat), 39 mg cholesterol, 502 mg sodium, 11 g carbohydrates, 5 g fiber, 3 g sugars (0 g added sugars), 31 g protein*

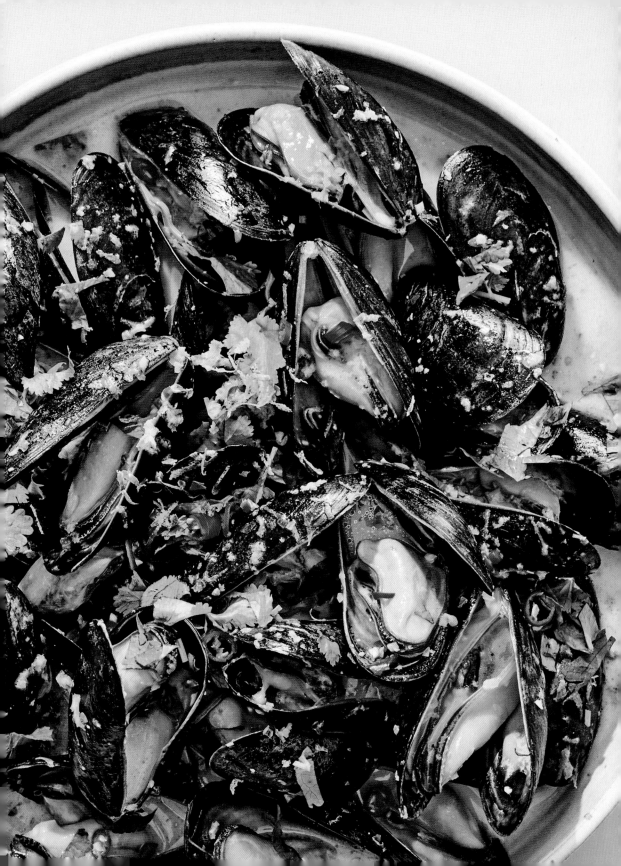

Lemongrass Coconut Mussels

TOTAL 15 MIN. **SERVES** 4

2 Tbsp oil

2 large cloves garlic, finely chopped

1 stalk lemongrass, trimmed and finely chopped

1 small red chile, thinly sliced, plus more for serving

2 tsp grated fresh ginger

1 13.5-oz can unsweetened regular or light coconut milk, well shaken

2 tsp fish sauce

3 lbs mussels, scrubbed, beards removed

1 tsp lime zest plus 1 Tbsp juice

¾ cup cilantro leaves

Crusty bread

1. Heat oil, garlic, and lemongrass in Dutch oven on medium-low until sizzling and fragrant, about 3 min.

2. Stir in chile and ginger, cook 1 min., then add coconut milk and fish sauce. Bring mixture to a simmer, then add mussels. Cover and simmer, stirring once or twice, until shells open, 5 to 6 min.

3. Toss with lime zest and juice. Sprinkle with cilantro and chile and serve with bread.

Per serving About 466 calories, 33 g fat (19.5 g saturated fat), 67 mg cholesterol, 899 mg sodium, 14 g carbohydrates, 0 g fiber, 0.5 g sugars (0 g added sugars), 31 g protein

Test Kitchen Trick **TO CLEAN MUSSELS, rinse and scrub under cold water. Then remove the beard by grabbing the membrane and pulling downward towards the hinged end of the shell.**

Super Green Soup with Parm Crisps

TOTAL 1 HR. 10 MIN. **SERVES** 4

2 Tbsp pine nuts, roughly chopped

⅓ cup finely grated Parmesan

2 Tbsp olive oil

5 large shallots, chopped (2 to 3 cups)

6 large garlic cloves, smashed

Kosher salt and pepper

5 cups bone or vegetable broth

⅓ cup red lentils

1½ tsp freshly grated nutmeg

2 large bunches spinach (about 14 oz), thick stems removed (10 to 12 cups)

1½ cup flat-leaf parsley leaves

1. Heat medium nonstick skillet on medium. Add pine nuts and cook, tossing, until toasted, 2 to 3 min.; transfer to small bowl. Sprinkle Parmesan in 7- to 8-inch round iron skillet, sprinkle with pine nuts, and cook until golden brown, about 5 min. Remove from heat and let cook until slightly crisp, 45 seconds to 1 min. Pry up edges and transfer to plate to cool completely, then break into shards.

2. Heat oil in medium saucepan on medium-low. Add shallots, garlic, and 1 tsp salt and cook, stirring occasionally, until beginning to soften, 6 min. Stir in broth, lentils, and ½ tsp pepper and bring to a boil. Reduce heat and gently simmer, covered, stirring occasionally, until lentils are just tender, 15 to 20 min.

3. Return to a boil, and stir in nutmeg and half of spinach, and return to a boil. Stir in remaining spinach and parsley leaves, then immediately blend in batches until smooth.

4. Cool any soup for future use over an ice bath. Serve soup with Parmesan crisps sprinkled on top.

Per serving *About 337 calories, 12.5 g fat (2.5 g saturated fat), 25 g protein, 1,026 mg sodium, 36 g carbohydrates, 8.5 g sugars (0 g added sugars), 8 g fiber*

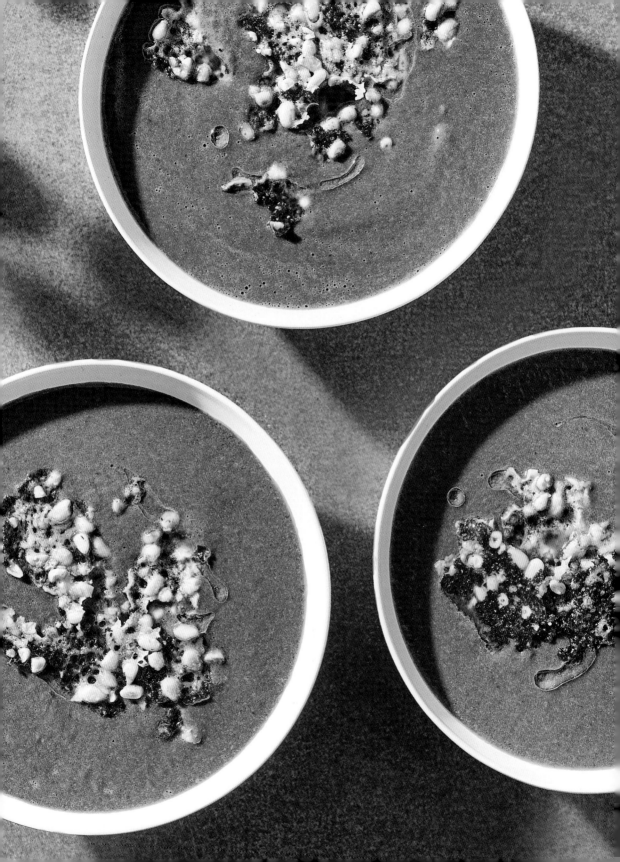

Vegan Mac and Cheese

TOTAL 30 MIN. **SERVES** 4

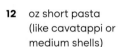

12	oz short pasta (like cavatappi or medium shells)
⅓	cup panko bread crumbs
1	Tbsp plus 2 tsp olive oil
¼	cup fresh parsley, finely chopped, divided
1	small onion, finely chopped
	Kosher salt and pepper
2	cloves garlic, pressed
1	cup cashews
¼	tsp mustard powder or 1 tsp Dijon
	Pinch of cayenne
⅓	cup nutritional yeast

1. Heat oven to 425°F. Cook pasta per package directions; drain and transfer back to pot. In small bowl, combine panko with 2 tsp oil and spread on baking sheet and roast until golden brown; toss with parsley.

2. Heat remaining Tbsp oil in small saucepan on medium. Add onion and ½ tsp each salt and pepper and cook covered, stirring occasionally until tender, 8 min. Stir in garlic and cook 1 min. Remove from heat and stir in cashews, mustard powder, and cayenne. Add 1½ cups water and bring mixture to a boil. Reduce heat and simmer until cashews are tender, 10 to 12 min.

3. Transfer mixture to blender, add nutritional yeast and ½ cup water, and puree until smooth.

4. Transfer mixture back to saucepan and cook, stirring occasionally until thickened, 6 to 8 min.

5. Toss with pasta and serve sprinkled with parsley crumbs.

Per serving About 597 calories, 20 g fat (3.5 g saturated fat), 0 mg cholesterol, 266 mg sodium, 83 g carbohydrates, 7 g fiber, 5 g sugar (0 g added sugar), 23 g protein

POWER UP!
Nutritional yeast is complete plant protein that adds nutty and savory flavor. Sprinkle it on popcorn, pasta, roasted vegetables, or salads.

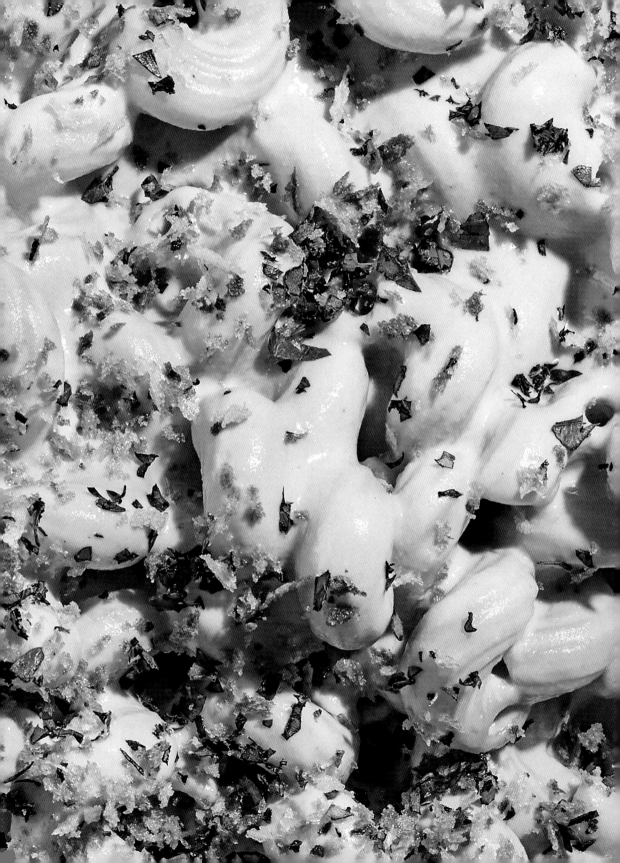

Creamy Chicken and Zoodle Spaghetti

TOTAL 30 MIN. **SERVES** 4

8 oz spaghetti

2½ Tbsp olive oil, divided

1 lb boneless, skinless chicken breasts, cut into 2-in. pieces

½ tsp Italian seasoning

Kosher salt and pepper

1 small shallot, finely chopped

1 clove garlic, finely chopped

½ cup dry white wine

½ cup sour cream

2 cup baby spinach

1 lb zucchini, spiralized

Grated lemon zest plus 1 Tbsp lemon juice

Grated Parmesan, for serving

1. Cook pasta per package directions. Drain, reserving ½ cup pasta water.

2. Heat 1 Tbsp oil in large deep-sided skillet on medium-high. Season chicken with Italian seasoning, ½ tsp salt, and ¼ tsp pepper; cook, turning occasionally, until golden brown all over, 5 to 7 min. Transfer to plate.

3. In same skillet, heat ½ Tbsp oil on medium. Add shallot and cook, stirring, until translucent, 1 min. Stir in garlic and cook until fragrant, 30 seconds. Add wine and simmer until reduced by half, 2 min. Whisk in sour cream and ¼ tsp salt.

4. Remove skillet from heat, add spaghetti, and toss, adding reserved pasta water 2 Tbsp at a time as needed, until saucy. Fold in spinach to wilt (return to heat as necessary).

5. Meanwhile, in large bowl, toss zoodles with lemon juice and remaining Tbsp oil until coated. Add pasta and toss to combine, then toss with chicken. Serve topped with lemon zest and Parmesan.

Per serving About 497 calories, 17.5 g fat (4.5 g saturated fat), 77 mg cholesterol, 451 mg sodium, 50 g carbohydrates, 4 g fiber, 5 g sugar (0 g added sugar), 34 g protein

Prep Ahead **YOU CAN MAKE** your zoodles with a spiralizer, a mandoline, or a julienne peeler. Store your zoodles in the fridge in a covered container lined with paper towels.

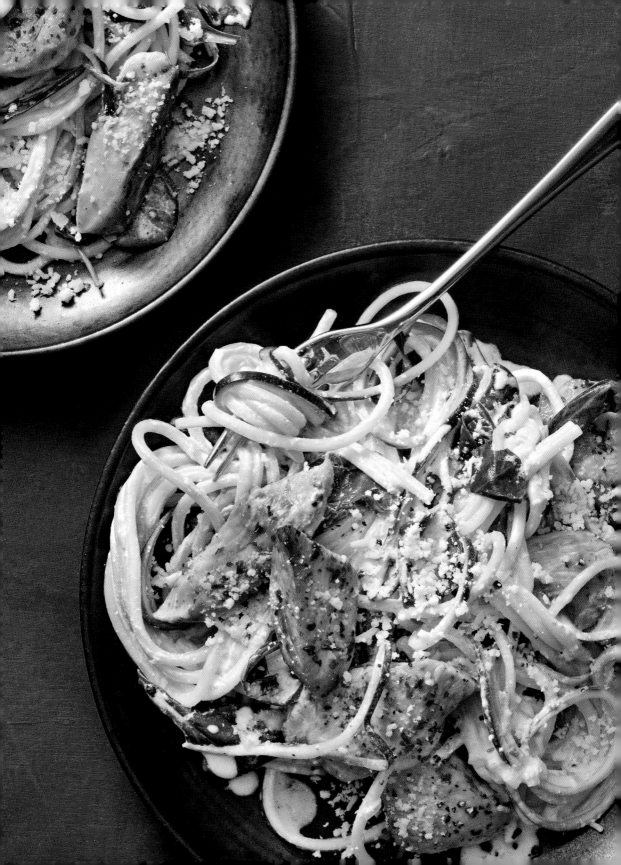

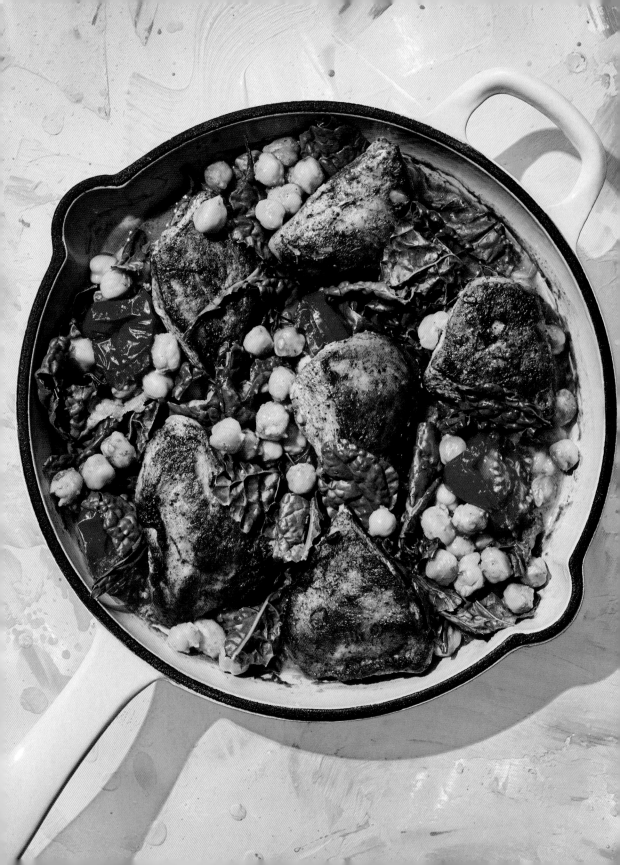

Skillet Chicken and Chickpeas

TOTAL 10 MIN. **SERVES** 4

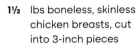

1½   lbs boneless, skinless chicken breasts, cut into 3-inch pieces

1½   tsp garam masala, divided

Kosher salt and pepper

1½   Tbsp olive oil, divided

2   cloves garlic, finely chopped

1   tsp grated fresh ginger

½   cup dry white wine

1   lb Campari tomatoes, halved crosswise

2   15-oz cans low-sodium chickpeas, 1 can rinsed, 1 can with liquid intact

8   oz lacinato kale, stems removed, leaves roughly chopped into 2-inch pieces (about 5 cups)

Cooked rice or crusty bread, for serving

1. Heat oven to 450°F. Pat chicken dry with paper towels, then season with 1 tsp garam masala and ¼ tsp salt.

2. Heat ½ Tbsp oil in large oven-safe skillet on medium and cook chicken on one side until deep golden brown, 5 to 6 min. Flip chicken, add garlic and ginger, and drizzle with remaining Tbsp oil; cook 1 min., then season with ¼ tsp each salt and pepper and remaining ½ tsp garam masala.

3. Add wine and bring to a simmer, scraping browned bits from bottom of pan; cook until liquid reduces slightly, 3 to 4 min. Add tomatoes and chickpeas (along with liquid from 1 can) and simmer, 3 min. (Tomatoes will release some liquid.)

4. Transfer skillet to oven and roast 8 min. Add kale, cover, and return to oven until chicken is cooked through and kale wilts slightly, 3 min. Remove from oven, gently toss ingredients, and let stand 3 min. Serve with rice or crusty bread.

Per serving *About 388 calories, 11 g fat (1.5 g saturated fat), 99 mg cholesterol, 485 mg sodium, 32 g carbohydrates, 9 g fiber, 7 g sugar (1.5 g added sugar), 41 g protein*

Test Kitchen Trick   **PATTING CHICKEN DRY before** cooking **removes excess moisture that prevents browning.**

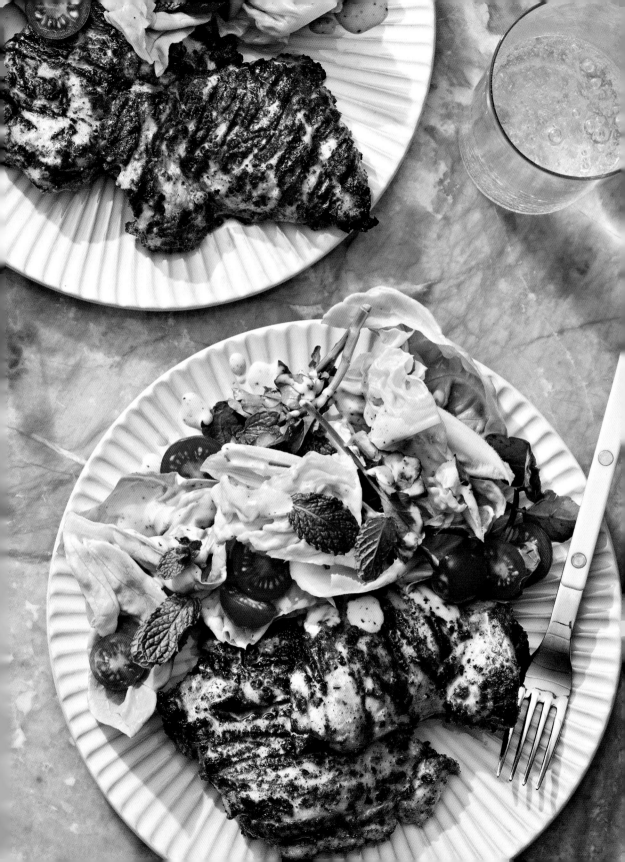

Lemon Tahini–Marinated Chicken

TOTAL 25 MIN. **SERVES** 4

1 cup tahini

2 tsp finely grated lemon zest plus 1½ Tbsp lemon juice

2 tsp honey

1 tsp sumac

2 cloves garlic, grated

Kosher salt and pepper

8 small boneless, skinless chicken thighs (about 2 lbs)

1 Tbsp olive oil, plus more for brushing grill

6 cups salad greens

2 Persian cucumbers, quartered and chopped

¼ pint grape tomatoes, halved

¼ cup mint leaves, torn

1. In large bowl, whisk tahini, lemon zest, honey, sumac, garlic, ½ tsp salt, and ¼ tsp pepper until smooth. Remove ¼ cup and set aside.
2. Add chicken to remaining tahini mixture and turn chicken to coat completely. Let marinate at least 1 hr. or transfer to resealable plastic bag and refrigerate overnight.
3. Heat grill to medium and brush grates with oil. Grill chicken until instant-read thermometer registers 165°F, 7 to 8 min. per side (discard marinade from bag).
4. Meanwhile, in large bowl, whisk together reserved tahini mixture, lemon juice, 2 Tbsp water, and oil.
5. Arrange salad greens, cucumbers, tomatoes, and chicken on platter. Drizzle with tahini dressing and sprinkle with mint.

Per serving *About 625 calories, 40.5 g fat (7.5 g saturated fat), 208 mg cholesterol, 378 mg sodium, 24 g carbohydrates, 8 g fiber, 4.5 g sugar (1.5 g added sugar), 49 g protein*

POWER UP!
Tahini is a paste made from ground sesame seeds that's popular in Mediterranean dishes. One tablespoon offers 3 grams of protein.

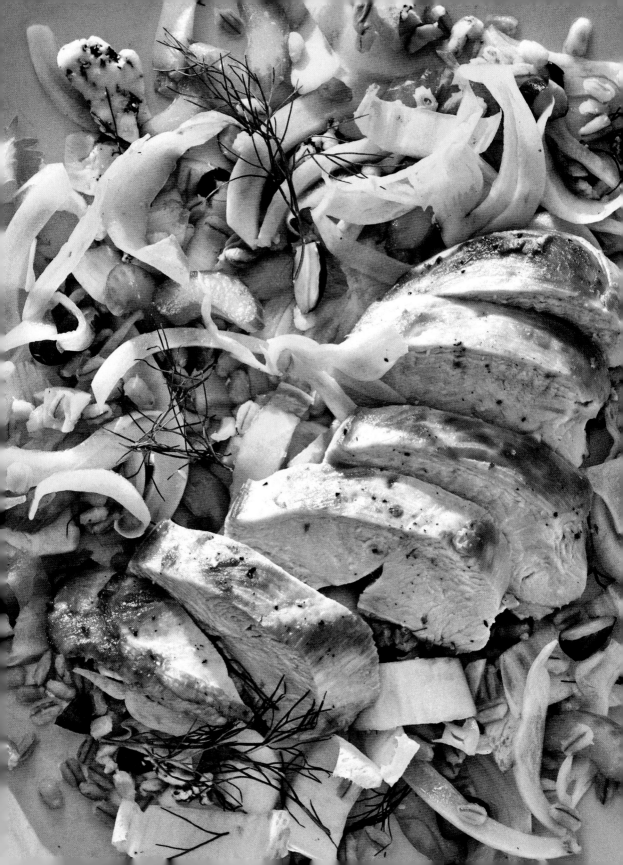

Endive Salad with Chicken and Blue Cheese

TOTAL 40 MIN. **SERVES** 4

1 cup barley

5 Tbsp olive oil, divided

4 5-oz boneless, skinless chicken breasts

Kosher salt and pepper

3 Tbsp fresh lemon juice, divided

2 heads endive, sliced crosswise ½ in.-thick

1 medium fennel-bulb, very thinly sliced, plus ¼ cup fennel fronds

3 ribs celery, thinly sliced on bias, plus ¼ cup celery leaves

1 oz blue cheese, crumbled

¼ cup roasted salted almonds, chopped

1. Cook barley per package directions. Rinse with cold water until cool, then drain thoroughly.

2. Meanwhile, heat 1 Tbsp oil in large skillet on medium. Season chicken with ½ tsp salt and ¼ tsp pepper. Cook in single layer, adjusting heat as needed to prevent burning, until deep golden brown and cooked through, 6 to 7 min. per side.

3. Remove from heat and drizzle with 1 Tbsp lemon juice. Transfer to cutting board and let rest at least 3 min. before slicing.

4. In large bowl, whisk remaining 4 Tbsp oil and 2 Tbsp lemon juice with ¼ tsp each salt and pepper. Add cooked barley, endive, sliced fennel, and celery ribs and toss to combine.

5. Serve chicken with salad sprinkled with blue cheese, almonds, fennel fronds, and celery leaves.

Per serving *About 446 calories, 25.5 g fat (5 g saturated fat), 84 mg cholesterol, 690 mg sodium, 21 g carbohydrates, 6 g fiber, 3.5 g sugar (0 g added sugar), 34 g protein*

Test Kitchen Trick **LOOK FOR** pearled barley, which doesn't require soaking before cooking.

Kale Chicken Salad

TOTAL 25 MIN. **SERVES** 4

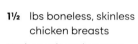

1½ lbs boneless, skinless chicken breasts

Kosher salt and pepper

2 lemons, halved

2 thick slices country bread

1 clove garlic, halved, plus ½ small clove garlic, finely grated

1 large egg yolk

½ tsp Dijon mustard

¼ cup olive oil

¼ cup grated Parmesan

5 oz baby kale

1. Cut chicken into 1½-inch chunks; thread onto skewers and season with ¼ tsp each salt and pepper. Grill, turning occasionally, until cooked through, 6 to 8 min.
2. Grill 1 lemon half, cut-side down, until charred; squeeze over chicken. Grill bread until toasted, rub both sides with garlic halves, then cut into pieces.
3. From remaining lemon, finely grate 1 tsp zest and squeeze 4 Tbsp juice into bowl. Whisk in yolk, mustard, grated garlic, and ½ tsp salt. Whisk in oil. Fold in Parmesan, kale, and croutons. Serve with chicken.

Per serving *About 424 calories, 20.5 g fat (4.5 g saturated fat), 86 g cholesterol, 707 mg sodium, 18 g carbohydrates, 1 g sugars (0 g added sugars), 2 g fiber, 41 g protein*

POWER UP!

Baby kale is the term for the young, tender leaves of a hearty plant. It's a nutritional powerhouse, rich in vitamins A, C, and K, as well as calcium and iron.

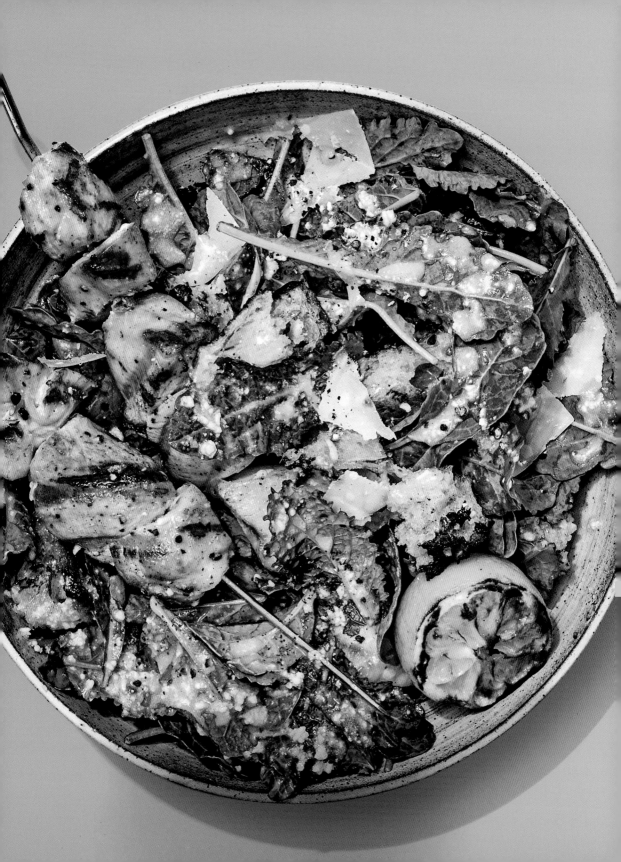

Crispy Parmesan Tofu Cutlets

TOTAL 45 MIN. **SERVES** 4

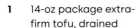

1	14-oz package extra-firm tofu, drained
2	Tbsp olive oil, divided
2	large eggs
3	cloves garlic, grated, divided

Kosher salt and black pepper

¾	cup grated Parmesan
¼	cup all-purpose flour
1½	Tbsp lemon juice
1	lb mixed cherry tomatoes, halved
½	cup basil leaves, roughly chopped
2	cups watercress

1. Heat oven to 400°F. Slice tofu into 8 equal pieces (each about ⅓-inch thick). Place on cutting board between paper towels; top with a baking sheet. Top with large cans or other weights and let stand 10 min.

2. Line baking sheet with parchment paper and rub with 1 Tbsp oil. In shallow bowl, whisk together eggs, 2 cloves grated garlic, and ½ tsp each salt and pepper. Place half Parmesan in second shallow bowl and flour in third bowl.

3. Halve each piece tofu into a triangle, dip in flour, then egg, letting excess drip off, and finally in Parmesan, pressing gently to help it adhere, and place on prepared sheet (add remaining Parmesan to bowl as needed). Roast until golden brown and crisp, 12 to 18 min. per side.

4. Meanwhile, in large bowl, whisk together lemon juice, remaining Tbsp oil, remaining grated garlic, and ½ tsp each salt and pepper. Toss with tomatoes and basil and let sit. Just before serving, toss with watercress and serve with tofu.

Per serving 256 calories, 10.5 g fat (2 g saturated fat), 95 mg cholesterol, 476 mg sodium, 32 g carbohydrates, 3 g fiber, 15 g sugar (0 g added sugar), 11 g protein

POWER UP!
Tofu—made from curdling soy milk and forming it into a solid block— is a great vegan protein option.

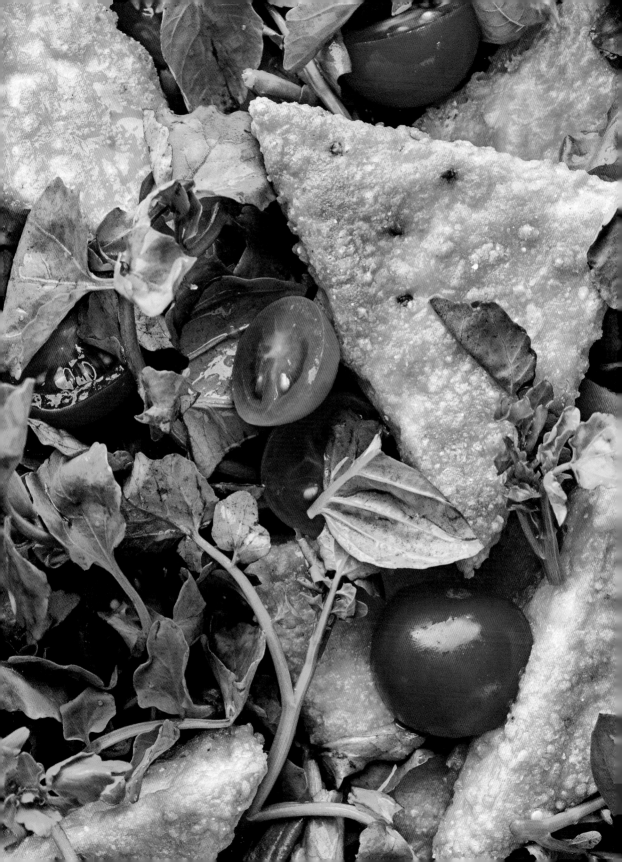

Gochujang Steak Salad with Sugar Snaps and Radishes

TOTAL 30 MIN. SERVES 4

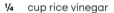

¼ cup rice vinegar

2 Tbsp olive oil

2 Tbsp gochujang paste

1 Tbsp reduced-sodium soy sauce

Pinch of sugar

1 lb beef flank steak

Kosher salt and pepper

8 oz snap peas, thinly sliced on bias (about 2 cups)

½ seedless cucumber, thinly sliced

6 radishes, thinly sliced

2 scallions, thinly sliced

1 head butter or Bibb lettuce, torn into pieces (about 8 cups)

Crushed peanuts, for serving (optional)

1. Heat grill to medium-high. In bowl, whisk together vinegar, oil, gochujang paste, soy sauce, and sugar. Transfer 2 Tbsp dressing to large bowl; set aside.

2. Season steak with ¼ tsp each salt and pepper and grill 5 min. Flip steak and cook to desired doneness, 4 to 5 min. more, basting with dressing during last 3 min. of grilling. Transfer to cutting board and let rest at least 5 min. before slicing.

3. In same large bowl with dressing, toss snap peas, cucumber, radishes, scallions, and lettuce. Fold in beef and any remaining dressing and sprinkle with peanuts, if desired.

Per serving *About 302 calories, 15 g fat (4 g saturated fat), 68 g cholesterol, 572 mg sodium, 14 g carbohydrates, 8 g sugars (<1 g added sugars), 3 g fiber, 27 g protein*

 Test Kitchen Trick GOCHUJANG spice level varies so make sure you check the package label.

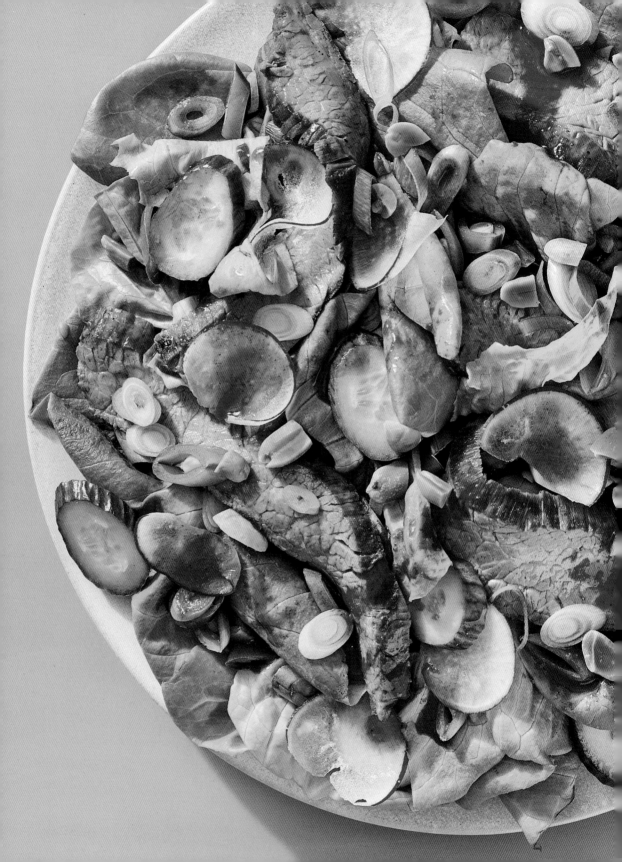

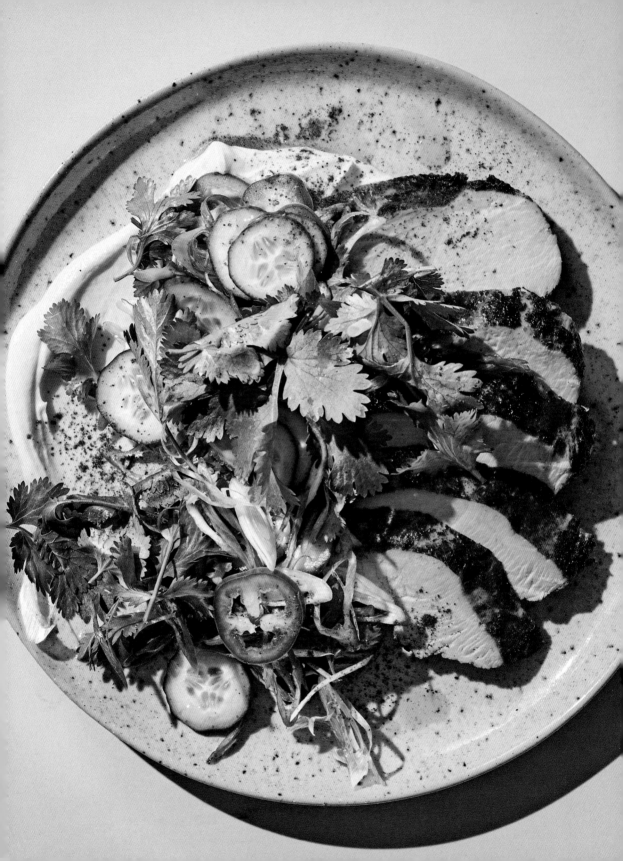

Shawarma-Spiced Chicken with Cucumber Salad

TOTAL 30 MIN. **SERVES** 4

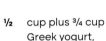

½ cup plus ¾ cup Greek yogurt, divided

2 Tbsp fresh lemon juice

2 Tbsp shawarma seasoning

1 large clove garlic, grated

Kosher salt

4 6-oz boneless, skinless chicken breasts

1 olive oil, plus more for drizzling

2 Persian cucumbers, thinly sliced

4 scallions, thinly sliced

1 jalapeño, thinly sliced

1 cup cilantro leaves

1. In medium bowl, combine ½ cup Greek yogurt with lemon juice, then shawarma seasoning, garlic, and ½ tsp salt. Add chicken and coat thoroughly. Let marinate 5 min.

2. Remove chicken from marinade, pat dry, and season with ¼ tsp salt. Heat oil in large cast-iron skillet on medium and cook chicken, adjusting heat as needed to prevent burning, until deep golden brown and cooked through, 6 to 7 min. per side. Transfer to cutting board and let rest at least 3 min. before slicing.

3. Meanwhile, in another bowl, toss together cucumbers, scallions, jalapeño, and then cilantro.

4. Divide remaining ¾ cup yogurt among plates. Top with sliced chicken and salad. Drizzle with additional oil.

Per serving *About 276 calories, 10 g fat (3 g saturated fat), 100 mg cholesterol, 273 mg sodium, 6 g carbohydrates, 1 g fiber, 3 g sugar (0 g added sugar), 39 g protein*

Test Kitchen Trick SHAWARMA is an earthy Middle Eastern spice blend that contains warming spices like cinnamon, coriander, cardamom, and tumeric.

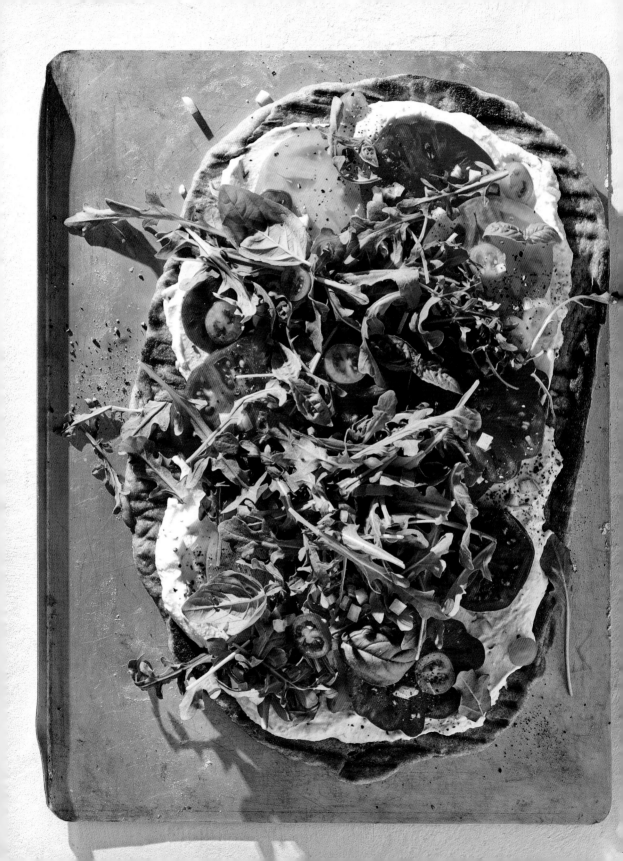

"Caprese" Pizza

TOTAL 25 MIN. **SERVES** 4

Prepared whole-wheat pizza dough, at room temp for 1 hr. if refrigerated

¾ cup whole-milk cottage cheese

1 oz Parmesan, finely grated (⅔ cup), plus more for sprinkling

¼ cup basil leaves, chopped, plus more for sprinkling

1 tsp lemon zest, plus 1 Tbsp lemon juice

3 medium heirloom tomatoes, sliced

½ cup cherry tomatoes

1 Tbsp olive oil

½ tsp honey

Kosher salt and pepper

1 small shallot, chopped

4 cups baby arugula

1. Grill pizza dough (instructions below); transfer to a cutting board.

2. In food processor puree cottage cheese until smooth, then pulse in Parmesan. Transfer to bowl and fold in basil and lemon zest. Spread cheese mixture onto pizza crust and top with tomatoes.

3. In large bowl, whisk together oil, lemon juice, honey, ¼ tsp salt, and ⅛ tsp pepper to dissolve; stir in shallot. Add arugula and toss to coat. Top tomatoes with arugula salad and sprinkle with additional Parmesan, if desired.

Per serving *About 468 calories, 21 g fat (4.5 g saturated fat), 10 mg cholesterol, 842 mg sodium, 49 g carbohydrates, 9 g fiber, 9 g sugar (3.5 g added sugar), 19 g protein*

How to Grill Pizza Dough

1. Heat grill to medium-high and prepare one side for direct heat and other side for indirect heat.

2. Working on floured surface, shape 1 lb pizza dough (at room temp, if refrigerated) into 12 to 14-inch round and transfer to flour-dusted baking sheet. Brush top with 2 tsp olive oil.

3. Grill dough, oiled side down, over direct heat, covered, until top begins to bubble and bottom is crisp, 2 to 4 min. (use tongs to peek underneath).

4. Brush top of dough with 2 tsp olive oil.

5. Flip dough and grill over indirect heat, then top as desired. Grill, covered, until crust is cooked through and charred on bottom, 3 to 5 min. (any cheese will melt during this time).

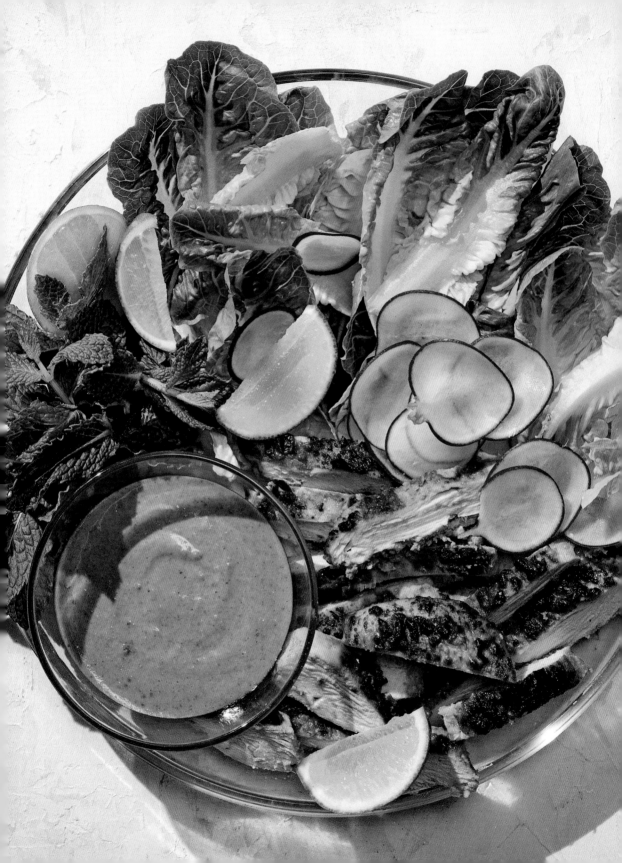

Chicken Lettuce Wraps with Sunbutter Dressing

TOTAL 45 MIN. **SERVES** 4

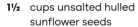

1½ cups unsalted hulled sunflower seeds

¼ cup shelled hemp seeds

1 to 3 tsp avocado oil

½ cup light coconut milk

3 Tbsp honey

2 Tbsp Thai red curry paste

1 Tbsp fish sauce

2 tsp lime zest plus 2 Tbsp juice

1 2-inch piece ginger, peeled and grated (about 1 Tbsp)

4 cloves garlic, grated

4 6-oz boneless, skinless chicken breasts, pounded to ½-inch thick

Kosher salt

2 heads little gem lettuce, leaves separated

4 radishes, thinly sliced

½ cup mint leaves

1. Heat oven to 375°F. Spread sunflower seeds on rimmed baking sheet and bake until toasted and fragrant, 10 to 12 min.; transfer to food processor (make sure it is dry). Add hemp seeds and process, scraping sides as needed, until smooth paste forms, 8 to 10 min. If too thick, add oil 1 tsp at a time until desired consistency is reached.

2. Add coconut milk, honey, curry paste, fish sauce, lime zest, and ginger; process until smooth, scraping sides as needed. Remove ½ cup to small bowl and set aside; transfer remaining to resealable bag and add garlic and chicken. Massage to coat. Let sit at room temp 15 min.

3. Meanwhile, heat broiler and arrange oven rack 6 in. from broiler. To reserved sauce, whisk in lime juice, ⅛ tsp salt, and 1 to 2 Tbsp water until pourable.

4. Place marinated chicken, nicer side up, on foil-lined baking sheet; broil until cooked through, 6 to 7 min. Transfer to cutting board and let rest 5 min. before slicing. Serve sliced chicken with lettuce, radishes, mint, and sunbutter dressing.

Per serving *About 677 calories, 40 g fat (6 g saturated fat), 94 mg cholesterol, 996 mg sodium, 32 g carbohydrates, 7 g fiber, 16.5 g sugar (13 g added sugar), 51 g protein*

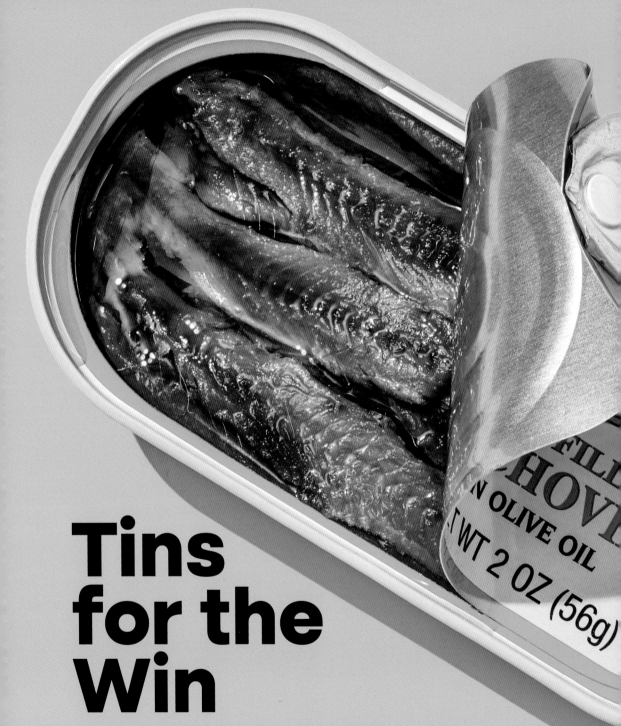

Tins for the Win

There may be plenty of fish in the sea, but these tiny containers are clutch for a convenient and affordable protein boost.

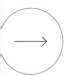

Tinned fish (also called canned fish) packs a ton of protein and deliciousness into tiny shelf-stable cans. While it's nothing new—fisheries were canning seafood as a preservation method well before refrigeration and freezing became common—the process remains incredibly relevant (and popular!) today.

The best tinned fish is full of flavor: Rather than only water-packed canned tuna, many brands are now serving up fillets packed in high-quality olive oil as well as seasonings like dried herbs, garlic, and spices. Tins also tend to be less expensive than their fresh counterparts. And while tinned fish, like fresh, is also ultra high in protein, it's a lot easier to keep a few cans in your pantry for a quick protein fix.

Canned fish boasts benefits beyond convenience and cost; it's really good for you too. "Eating one to two 3-ounce servings of fatty fish a week may reduce the risk for heart attack, stroke, depression, Alzheimer's disease, and other chronic conditions," says Keri Glassman, RD, CDN, a member of the *Women's Health* Advisory Board and founder of Nutritious Life and the Nutritious Life Studio.

How to shop for tinned fish

When scanning options, it's important to consider environmental impacts in the fishing process. More than one-third of the world's fisheries are overfished, leading to climate concerns, per the United Nations.

One thing to consider when reading the label: "Look for the Marine Stewardship Council certification on cans," says Rebecca Goldburg, PhD, director of environmental research and science at The Pew Charitable Trusts.

If you're worried about mercury, the much-talked-about metal, good news: Many tins contain small fish, which have lower levels of mercury than big fish, per the FDA.

Sardines, mackerel, and shellfish, among others, don't feast on the fish that larger tuna or swordfish do, leaving them less susceptible to high levels of absorption. When buying tuna, look for skipjack varieties or those that rely on pole-and-line catching (a sustainable sourcing method).

Best tinned fish recipe ideas

Not sure what to serve with tinned fish? It can be as simple as pairing open cans with crackers, tossing into salads, topping toasts, or folding into wraps for a simple protein- packed lunch. Tinned fish is so versatile, and because it's already cooked, it makes a great addition to no-cook recipes.

Top toast

Add mackerel to avocado toast (shout out to a high-protein breakfast), pile sourdough high with flaky smoked trout, or dot anchovies across an egg-topped crusty bread. Oily tinned fish pairs nicely with really any slice, so get creative!

Build an incredible charcuterie board

Try cracking open a few cans, adding pickles, crackers, and crunchy veggies to make a pescatarian charcuterie board (lazy dinner, ftw!) where the whole family can build their own bite. Or it makes a genius appetizer for any party.

Serve a better salad

If you're looking to boost protein in your go-to lunch (or dinner!) salad, flaking tinned fish and tossing with veggies is a great way to do it.

Stir into sauces

These little fish can pack big flavor. Stir tinned fish like salmon, skipjack, or tuna into a prepared pasta sauce or blend anchovies into a salad dressing.

Rotisserie Rockstar

One of the simpliest hacks to eating more lean protein: this ready-made bird on your weekly shopping list.

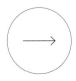

Why are rotisserie chickens so fantastic? To state the obvious, for starters, you can buy them at most grocery stores and big box stores already cooked so you can bring them home and eat them or prep them immediately. As for macros, one whole rotisserie chicken will generally give you about 4 cups of meat and around 165 grams of protein in total.

HOW TO BUY at the Store

▷ **Inspect it carefully.** When it sits under a heat lamp all day, the skin dries out and shrivels. The freshest birds will be plump and evenly browned.

▷ **Double check that it's hot, hot, hot.** Bacteria grow most rapidly between 40°F and 140°F, so grab the hottest chicken. Also: Make it the last item on your grocery list so it won't sit in the cart too long.

▷ **Feel the weight.** Rotisserie chickens tend to weigh around 2.5 pounds for consistent cooking. If a bird feels much lighter, that means more of its juices have evaporated, resulting in a drier bird.

▷ **Skip the flavored ones.** Specially seasoned birds are often higher in sodium. For the healthiest choice, opt for plain and then add salt and herbs at home.

WHAT TO DO at Home

▷ **Shred first, shred fast.** When you get home from the store, get to work! Shred the rotisserie chicken and/or remove the meat from the bones when it's still warm. (Otherwise, it'll get mushy if you wait until later.)

▷ **Bulk up a vegetable soup.** Take a can or box of something like butternut squash puree and add in shredded rotisserie chicken. Voila! Easy soothing protein-packed comfort dinner.

▷ **Wrap it in lettuce.** Whatever your favorite dressing and/or condiment, toss that with rotisserie chicken and you have an instant lettuce wrap filling. For example, try green goddess dressing mixed with shredded rotisserie chicken. Or mash guacamole with shredded chicken for an quick chicken salad.

▷ **Make a broth.** After you're done shredding and/or removing the meat, add the carcass to a slow cooker with onion, carrots, and celery along with parsley stems, thyme, or rosemary. Cover with water and let cook on low for 10 hours.

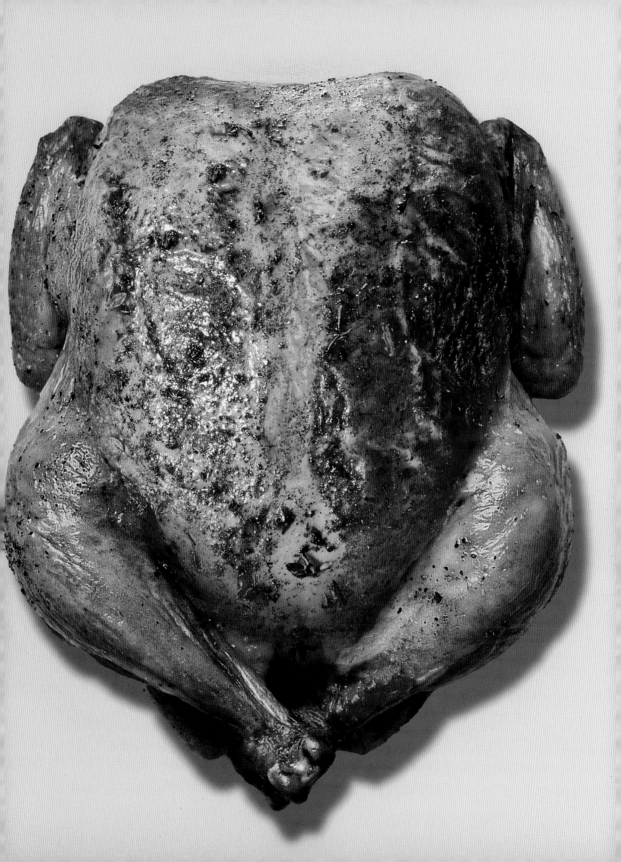

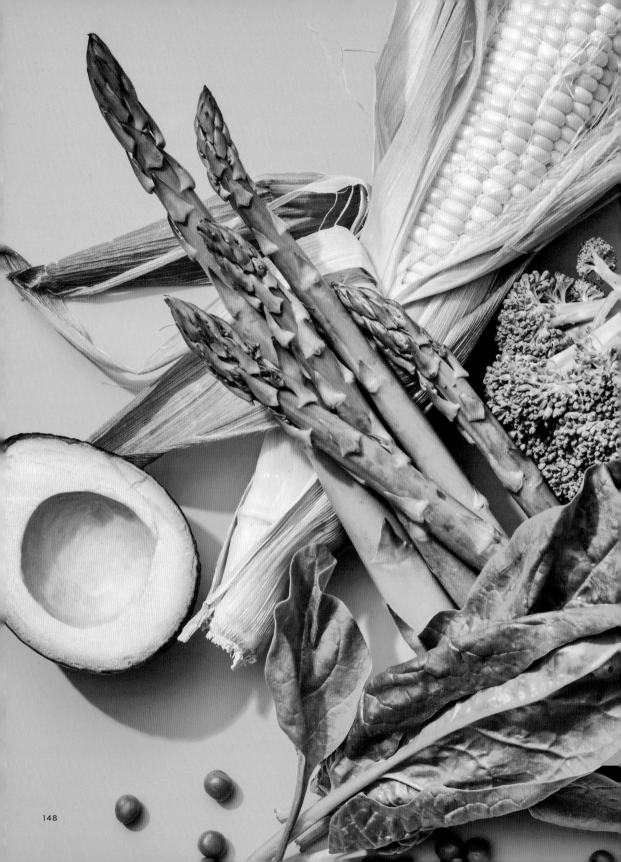

12 High-Protein Veggies That Will Fill You Up Fast

1. ARTICHOKE HEARTS
Artichoke hearts are also rich in potassium, fiber, and vitamin C.

Per ½-cup serving *45 calories, 0.3 g fat (0 g saturated), 10 g carbohydrates, 1 g sugar, 50 mg sodium, 4.8 g fiber, 2.5 g protein*

2. ASPARAGUS
In addition to vitamin C, asparagus is also a great source of fiber, plus you'll get some potassium and B vitamins too.

Per ½-cup serving *20 calories, 0.2 g fat (0 g saturated), 3.7 g carbohydrates, 1 g sugar, 12.6 mg sodium, 2 g fiber, 2.1 g protein.*

3. AVOCADO
If you're planning on making it a meal, give your avocado a boost with another protein source.

Per 1-cup serving *368 calories, 33 g fat (0 g saturated), 20 g carbohydrates, 1.5 g sugar, 16 mg sodium, 15 g fiber, 4.6 g protein*

4. BAKED POTATO
A medium-size baked potato also contains tons of vitamin C, potassium, and some filling fiber.

Per medium potato *145 calories, 0 g fat (0 g saturated), 34 g carbohydrates, 3 g sugar, 8 mg sodium, 2 g fiber, 3 g protein*

5. BROCCOLI
This cruciferous veggie isn't only packed with essential nutrients, fiber, and protein, it's great for maintaining proper gut health too.

Per 1-cup serving *31 calories, 0.3 g fat (0 g saturated), 6 g carbohydrates, 2 g sugar, 30 mg sodium, 2 g fiber, 3 g protein*

6. BROCCOLI RABE
Also known as "rapini," broccoli rabe (pronounced "rob") also contains vitamin A and vitamin K.

Per 85 g serving *21 calories, 0 g fat (0 g saturated), 3 g carbohydrates, 1 g sugar, 48 mg sodium, 2 g fiber, 3 g protein*

7. BRUSSELS SPROUTS
A great source of potassium, vitamin A, vitamin K, and fiber.

Per ½-cup serving *28 calories, 4 g fat (0 g saturated), 6 g carbohydrates, 1 g sugar, 16 mg sodium, 2 g fiber, 2 g protein*

8. CORN
The sweet corn we enjoy on the grill is considered a vegetable, not a grain. And a surprisingly protein-loaded one, at that.

Per medium ear *88 calories, 1.4 g fat (0 g saturated), 19 g carbohydrates, 6 g sugar, 15 mg sodium, 2 g fiber, 3 g protein*

9. LIMA BEANS
The combination of high fiber and high protein makes these legumes (in this case, a veggie too) a satiating, nutrient-filled powerhouse.

Per ½-cup serving *105 calories, 0 g fat (0 g saturated), 20 g carbohydrates, 1 g sugar, 13 mg sodium, 5 g fiber, 6 g protein*

10. PEAS
Loaded with vitamin A, a good source of potassium and fiber. Steam them and toss them into pasta, rice, or salads.

Per ½ cup serving *59 calories, 0.3 g fat (0 g saturated), 10 g carbohydrates, 4 g sugar, 4 mg sodium, 4 g protein*

11. PORTOBELLO MUSHROOMS
This vegetable is also high in fiber and loaded with antioxidants.

Per 100 g serving *32 calories, .3 g fat (0 g saturated), 5 g carbohydrates, 5 mg sodium, 2 g fiber, 2.75 g protein*

12. SPINACH
You'll get vitamin C, folic acid, and other B vitamins alongside all that protein.

Per ½- cup serving *21 calories, 0 g fat (0 g saturated), 3 g carbohydrates, 0 g sugar, 63 mg sodium, 2 g fiber, 3 g protein*

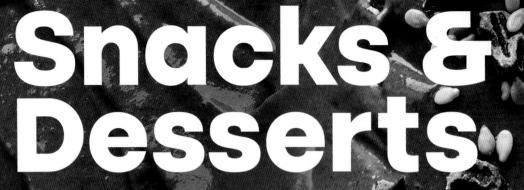

Snacks & Desserts

Need some oomph? Start here with small bites and sweet treats that are **big on flavor** and loaded with an energy boost.

Chocolate-Sesame Pudding

TOTAL 1½ HR. **SERVES** 4

5	oz Medjool dates, pitted
1	16-oz package silken tofu, drained
2	tsp pure vanilla extract
¼	tsp kosher salt
⅓	cup tahini
⅓	cup unsweetened cocoa powder
1	tsp toasted sesame seeds
1½	tsp cacao nibs

1. Microwave dates until warm, about 30 seconds, and place in blender. Add about half of tofu in blender along with vanilla and salt. Puree, scraping down sides as necessary, until as smooth as possible.

2. Add tahini, cocoa powder, and remaining tofu, and puree until incorporated.

3. Divide mixture among 4 small ramekins or bowls, jiggling slightly if you prefer a smooth surface, and refrigerate until set, 1 to 1½ hr. Top with sesame seeds and cacao nibs just before serving.

Per serving About 274 calories, 14 g fat (3 g saturatedfat), 0 mg cholesterol, 176 mg sodium, 37 g carbohydrates, 7 g fiber, 25 g sugar (0 g added sugar), 7 g protein

POWER UP!

Silken tofu boasts a, well, silky texture, plus a high moisture content, so it doubles for dairy this vegan dessert. To prep, avoid pressing since it will fall apart. Instead, cut into cubes.

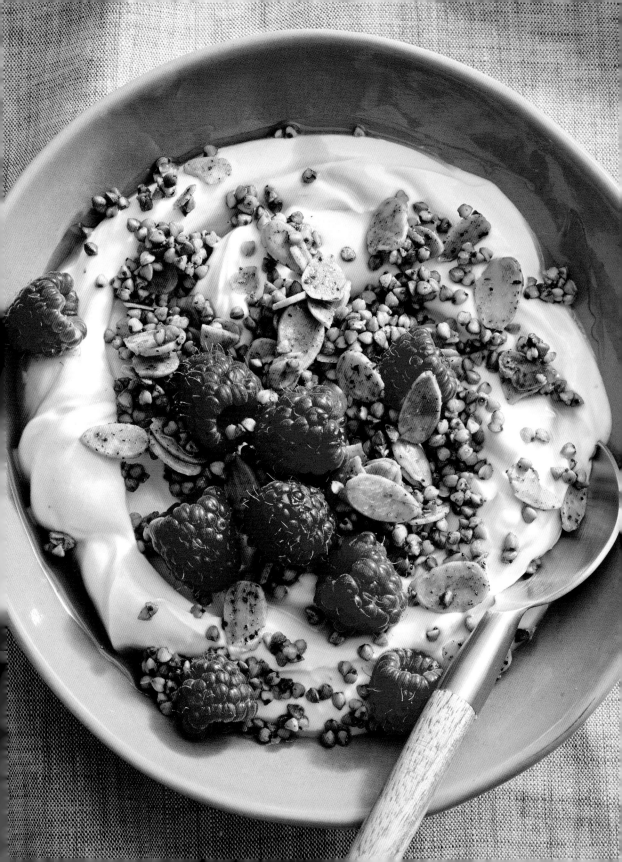

Yogurt with Strawberries and Almond-Buckwheat Groats

TOTAL 40 MIN. **SERVES** 4

1	Tbsp olive oil
1½	Tbsp pure maple syrup, divided
Kosher salt	
½	cup buckwheat groats
¼	tsp ground cinnamon
⅓	cup sliced almonds
1	lb strawberries, thickly sliced
3	cups Greek yogurt

1. Heat oven to 300°F. Line small, rimmed baking sheet with parchment paper. In bowl, whisk together oil, 1 Tbsp maple syrup, and ¼ tsp salt.
2. Heat medium cast-iron skillet on medium-high. Add groats and toast, shaking and tossing often and adjusting heat as needed, until color and aroma deepen and groats are crisp, 1 to 2 min.
3. Transfer to bowl with maple syrup and toss to coat (it will sizzle), then stir in cinnamon and almonds. Spread onto prepared baking sheet and bake, stirring halfway through and rotating baking sheet, until golden brown, 15 to 20 min. Let cool.
4. In bowl, toss berries with remaining ½ Tbsp maple syrup and pinch of salt; let sit 5 min. Spoon berries and juices over yogurt; top with groats. Store leftover groats in airtight container at room temp for up to 10 days.

Per serving About 332 calories, 17 g fat (5.5 g saturated fat), 25 mg cholesterol, 250 mg sodium, 27 g carbohydrates, 4 g fiber, 18 g sugars (4.5 g added sugar), 20 g protein

Test Kitchen Trick DO NOT ADD the cinnamon before the buckwheat. This prevents burning and the cinnamon turning bitter.

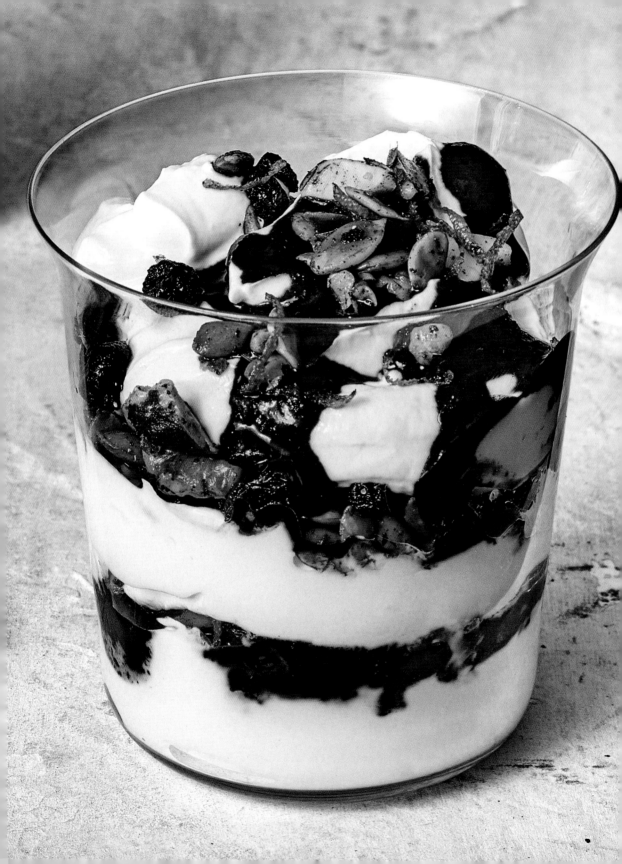

Blueberry-and-Mixed-Nut Parfait

TOTAL 35 MIN. **SERVES** 4

1	cup freeze-dried blueberries, divided
	Salt
3	Tbsp walnuts
3	Tbsp almonds
3	Tbsp pecans
3	Tbsp pepitas
1	Tbsp olive oil
1	tsp cinnamon
⅛	tsp cardamom
½	tsp flaky sea salt
1	Tbsp orange zest
¼	cup golden raisins
3	cups Greek yogurt

1. In food processor, pulse ½ cup freeze-dried blueberries to form a powder; transfer to small saucepan. Whisk in 1 cup water and simmer until thickened, about 15 min. Stir in pinch of salt; let sauce cool.

2. Meanwhile, toss walnuts, almonds, pecans, and pepitas with olive oil, cinnamon, cardamom, and flaky sea salt. Roast at 400°F until toasted, about 6 min., then toss with orange zest, remaining ½ cup freeze-dried blueberries, and golden raisins.

3. Make 4 parfaits, layering Greek yogurt (about ¾ cup each), blueberry sauce (about 1 heaping Tbsp), and nut mixture (heaping ¼ cup).

Per serving *About 415 calories, 25.5 g fat (6.5 g saturated fat), 25 mg cholesterol, 390 mg sodium, 28 g carbohydrates, 4 g fiber, 21.5 g sugar (0 g added sugar), 22 g protein*

POWER UP!
For other snack ideas that use Greek yogurt, turn to page 73.

Chocolate Protein Crispy Treats

TOTAL 10 MIN. **SERVES** 8

⅔ cup nut butter
of choice

½ cup honey or agave

2½ tsp pure vanilla
extract

¼ cup chocolate
protein powder

Salt

3 cups puffed rice
cereal (whole grain
or gluten free,
if desired)

2½ teaspoons pure
vanilla extract

Melted chocolate

Freeze-dried
strawberries

1. Mix nut butter, sweetener, vanilla, protein powder, and ½ tsp salt until smooth. Gently heat, then pour over cereal and stir very well, making sure to coat all of it.
2. Line pan with wax paper and spread mixture evenly into pan.
3. Place sheet of wax paper on top, then press down as firmly as you can. Really press it down!
4. Freeze for at least a half hr. before drizzling with chocolate, topping with strawberries, and slicing.

Per serving *About 273 calories, 14.5 g fat (3 g saturated fat), 6 mg cholesterol, 184 mg sodium, 32 g carbohydrates, 3 g fiber, 22 g sugar (17.5 g added sugar), 8 g protein*

Test Kitchen Trick **THERE ARE DOZENS** of types of nut butters to choose—from almond to cashew, peanut to walnut. Sometimes additional oils are added to the blends, but the more natural butters only contain the oils from the nuts and seeds themselves.

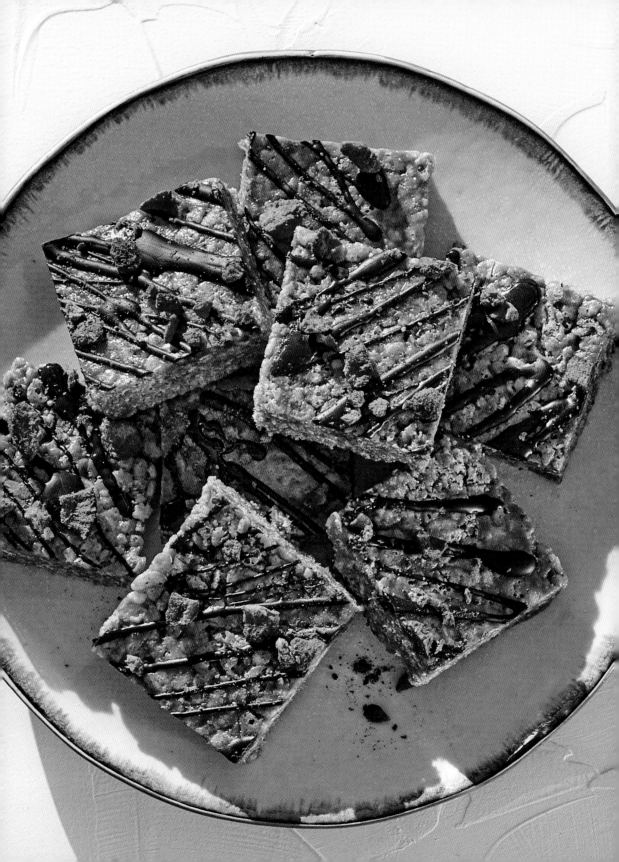

Mix-and-Match Protein Cookies

Choose Your Dough Base

VANILLA PROTEIN COOKIE DOUGH

In medium bowl, sift together ½ cup unflavored protein powder, ¾ cup oat flour, 1¼ cups almond meal, ½ tsp baking soda, and ¼ tsp salt; set aside. In large bowl, whisk together 6 Tbsp (¾ stick) melted butter, ¼ cup brown sugar, ¼ cup sugar, and ¼ cup almond butter. Whisk in 2 large eggs, one at a time, then 1 tsp vanilla extract. Add flour mixture and mix until fully incorporated.

CHOCOLATE PROTEIN COOKIE DOUGH

In medium bowl, sift together ½ cup chocolate protein powder, ½ cup Dutch-processed cocoa powder, ¼ cup oat flour, 1¼ cups almond meal, ½ tsp baking soda, and ¼ tsp salt. Set aside. In large bowl, whisk together 6 Tbsp (¾ stick) melted and cooled butter, ¼ cup brown sugar, ½ cup sugar, and ¼ cup almond butter. Whisk in 4 large eggs, one at a time, then 1 tsp vanilla extract. Add flour mixture and mix until fully incorporated.

Choose Your Mix-Ins

Pick a combo of crunchy, chewy, and sweet, but as long as you don't exceed 2½ cups total, you're golden! Fold in your mix-ins, then let dough sit to hydrate, covered with plastic wrap at room temp for 10 min. Some of our favorite combinations include:

Almond-Sunflower Seed

Vanilla Dough + 1½ cups natural almonds, sliced + 1 cup sunflower seeds

Apricot-Pecan

Vanilla Dough + 1½ cups dried apricots + 1 cup pecans

Cherry-Hazelnut

Vanilla Dough + 1½ cups dried cherries + 1 cup hazelnuts

Chocolate Pretzel-Banana

Chocolate Dough + 1 cup pretzels + 1 cup banana chips + ½ cup peanuts

Coconut Raisin

Vanilla Dough + 1 cup coconut flakes + 1½ cup golden raisins

Double Chocolate Sesame

Chocolate Dough + 1 cup cacao nibs + 1 cup sesame seeds + ½ cup puffed rice

Pistachio-Chocolate Chip

Vanilla Dough + 1 cup chocolate chips + 1 cup pistachios + ½ cup candied orange peels

Triple Chocolate and Strawberry

Chocolate Dough + 1 cup cacao nibs + 1 cup white chocolate chips + ½ cup freeze-dried strawberries

Bake the Cookies

Scoop ¼-cup mounds of dough (you should have about 24) and space them evenly on parchment-lined sheet trays. Press tops of cookies down to form flattened discs and bake at 350°F for 10 min. Rotate pan and bake until set around edges, about 3 min. more.

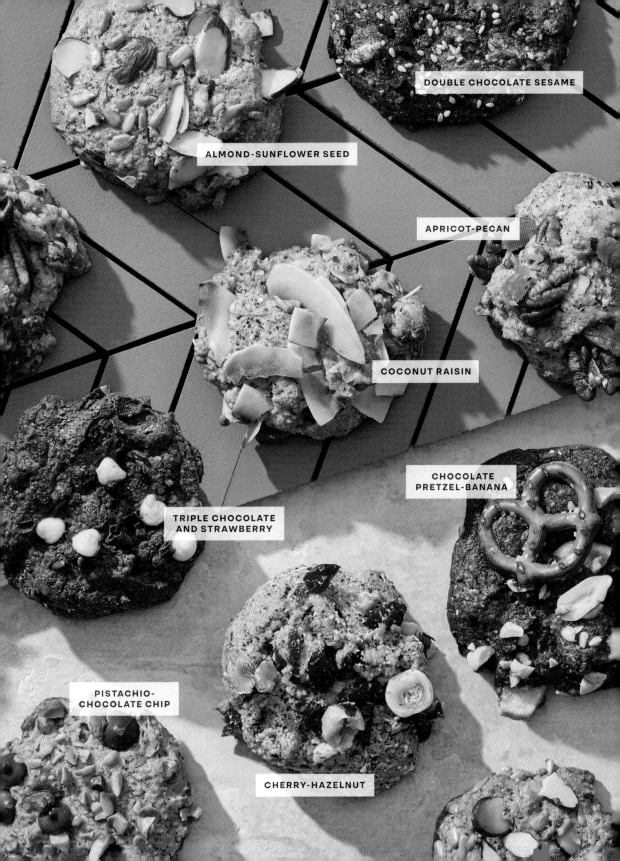

DOUBLE CHOCOLATE SESAME

ALMOND-SUNFLOWER SEED

APRICOT-PECAN

COCONUT RAISIN

CHOCOLATE
PRETZEL-BANANA

TRIPLE CHOCOLATE
AND STRAWBERRY

PISTACHIO-
CHOCOLATE CHIP

CHERRY-HAZELNUT

Spicy Salmon Nori Wraps

TOTAL 1 HR 20 MIN. **SERVES** 4

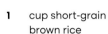

1	cup short-grain brown rice
3	Tbsp ponzu sauce
¼	tsp grated fresh ginger
3	Tbsp mayonnaise
2	Tbsp chili garlic sauce
2	6-oz cans boneless, skinless salmon, drained and flaked
8	sheets sushi nori
1	large scallion, thinly sliced
2	small Persian cucumbers, very thinly sliced
1½	tsp toasted sesame seeds

1. In small saucepan, combine rice with 1½ cups water. Bring to a vigorous simmer. Reduce heat, cover, and gently simmer, about 30 min. Remove from heat and let sit, covered, 5 min. Fluff with fork and let cool to room temp. Scoop out 1 cup (save remaining rice for other use).
2. In small bowl, combine ponzu and ginger; set aside. In medium bowl, combine mayonnaise and chili garlic sauce, then fold in salmon.
3. Lay out nori in 4 piles of 2 sheets each. Fold each pile into quarters, then unfold. Make a slit through each stack, starting from center and extending to bottom edge of nori, along middle crease, to create what will be a flap.
4. Working with 1 wrap at a time, on top left quadrant, arrange salmon mixture and top with scallions. Arrange cucumbers on top right quadrant. Using wet fingers, press brown rice onto bottom right quadrant, then top rice with sesame seeds.
5. Fold empty bottom left flap of nori up over salmon, then fold to the right, on top of cucumbers; finally, fold down over rice. Press gently to make it adhere and eat right away, drizzling with ponzu sauce.

Per serving About 269 calories, 12 g fat (2 g saturated fat), 63 mg cholesterol, 849 mg sodium, 18 g carbohydrates, 2 g fiber, 3.5 g sugar (3 g added sugar), 21 g protein

 Test Kitchen Trick **PONZU** is a Japanese dipping sauce known for its tangy, salty, citrus profile. It's made with soy sauce, vinegar, citrus juice, sugar, and mirin (rice wine).

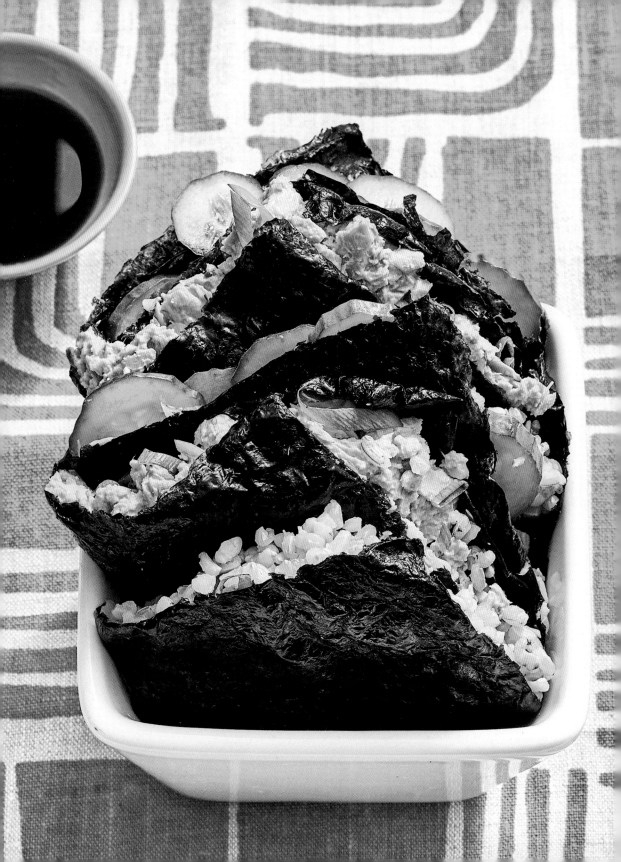

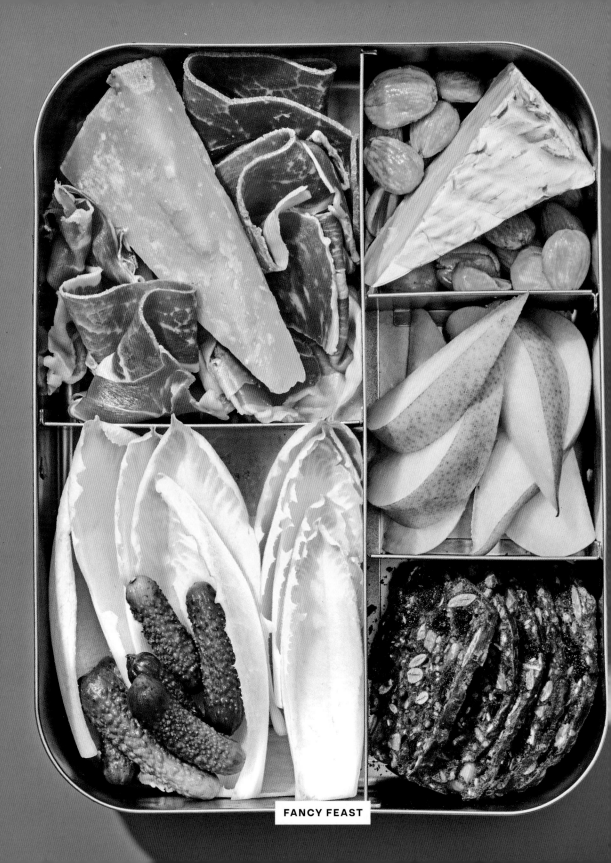

FANCY FEAST

How to Build a Protein-Packed
Snack Plate

For those days or nights when you don't feel like making
a full meal, may we suggest this quick and easy solution?

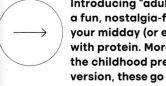

**Introducing "adult lunchables,"
a fun, nostalgia-filled way to pack
your midday (or end-of-day) meal
with protein. More elevated than
the childhood pre-packaged
version, these go beyond the typical
bologna, cheese "product," and salty crackers.**

These protein snack plates or protein boxes
have other benefits too: They're easy to assemble,
they offer tons of variety, and they can load in a
ton of protein with low-lift ingredients like sliced
turkey, canned tuna, hard-boiled eggs, and low-
sodium cheese.

You can meal prep and pack everything up
in a cute bento-style container the night before,
then take it to work and enjoy it all in one
go or graze on it at your whim. (Or prepare one
of these for dinner when you just don't feel
like cooking).

**The super-easy steps to build
a protein snack plate**

1. Start with a protein (and boost with more
protein, if you want).
2. Amp it up with some fiber (nuts, dried fruit).
3. Round it out with some fat to make it
satisfying (hello, cheese!).
4. Add fruit and raw veggies for crunch.
5. Complete the meal with healthy
crackers. The components are endlessly
customizable, so feel free to swap in your
faves for any of the recs.

Fancy Feast

- **PROTEIN** prosciutto + boost with
  thin Parm wedge
- **FIBER** Marcona almonds
- **FAT** triple-crème cheese, such as Brie
- **FRUIT** sliced pear
- **VEG** endive spears + cornichons
- **CRACKER** artisan nut and dried fruit crisps

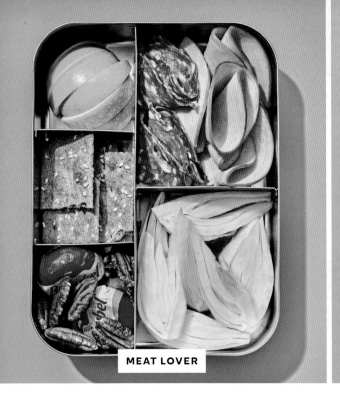

MEAT LOVER

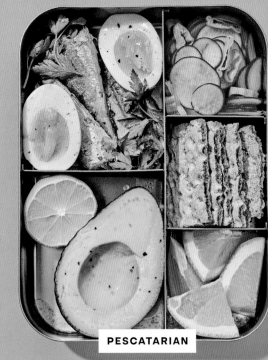

PESCATARIAN

Meat Lover

- **PROTEIN** sliced turkey + boost with another deli meat, like uncured soppressata
- **FIBER** pecans or your favorite nut
- **FAT** aged Gouda wedges or your favorite cheese
- **FRUIT** green apple wedges or your favorite fruit
- **VEG** fennel slices
- **CRACKER** stone-ground wheat crackers

Pescatarian

- **PROTEIN** canned tuna, salmon, or sardines + boost with hard-boiled egg
- **FIBER** avocado half with lemon
- **FAT** mayo to mix into fish (or prep tuna/salmon salad the night before)
- **FRUIT** Sumo citrus sections or your favorite citrus
- **VEG** radishes and pickled peppers
- **CRACKER** rye crispbread

Vegan

- **PROTEIN** hummus + boost with nut butter
- **FIBER** dried apricots, dates, or your favorite dried fruit
- **FAT** pistachios and chocolate
- **FRUIT** pomegranate seeds
- **VEG** sugar snap peas
- **CRACKER** lentil crackers

Vegetarian

- **PROTEIN** hard-boiled eggs + boost with cottage cheese
- **FIBER** sliced cukes
- **FAT** vegetarian chili crisp for drizzling + chocolate almond butter cup
- **FRUIT** grapes or your favorite fruit
- **VEG** cherry tomatoes
- **CRACKER** whole-grain crackers

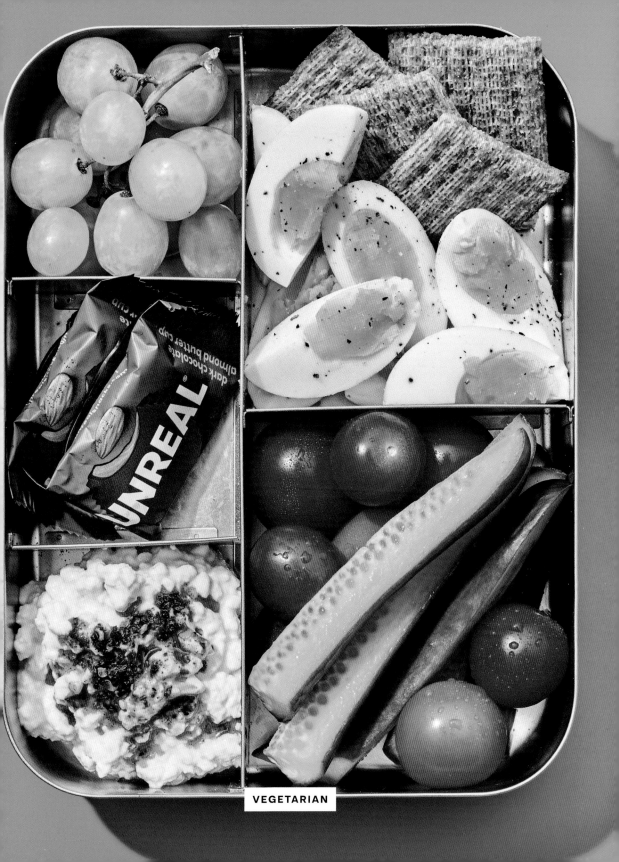

VEGETARIAN

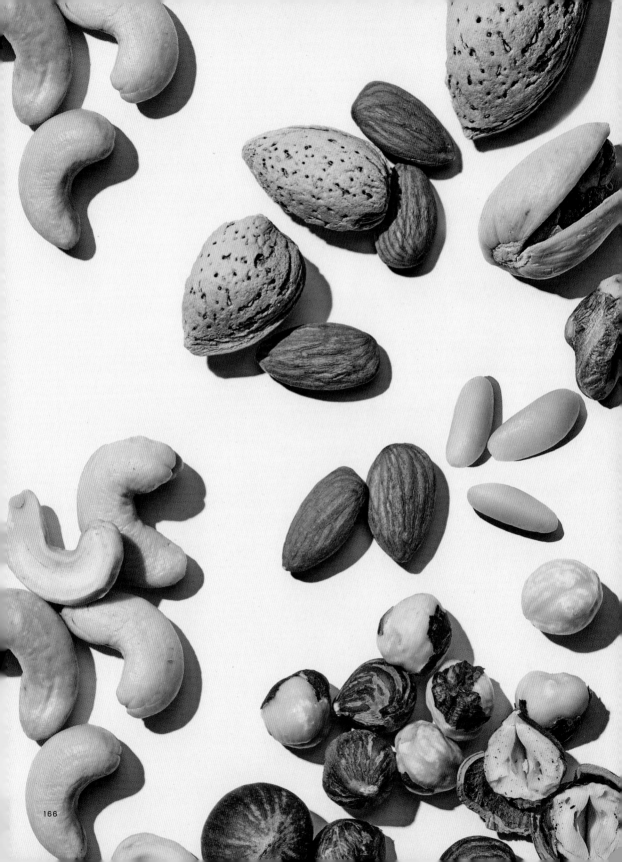

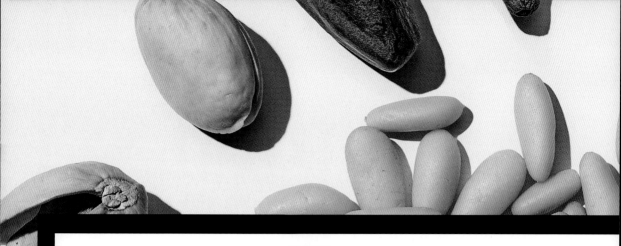

Go Nuts

Try these varieties for next-level snacking. (Psst: Keep a serving stashed in your bag for a protein boost if you get hangry.)

ALMONDS
Almonds also have bone-building calcium and antioxidants. Opt for skin-on almonds for a heap of fiber and an extra-nutty taste.

Per 1-oz serving *165 calories, 14 g fat (5 g saturated), 6 g carbs, 0 mg sodium, 0 g sugar, 3 g fiber, 6 g protein*

BRAZIL NUTS
Just one nut meets over 100 percent of the recommended daily allowance of selenium, a nutrient that helps protect against cell damage and infections.

Per 1-oz serving *186 calories, 19 g fat (4.5 g saturated), 3 g carbs, 0 mg sodium, 0 g sugar, 2 g fiber, 4 g protein*

CASHEWS
They're a triple-threat bundle of zinc, copper, and magnesium (which is great for immune support and muscle function), with a texture that makes a tasty stand-in for dairy.

Per 1-oz serving *157 calories, 12.5 g fat (2 g saturated), 9 g carbs, 0 mg sodium, 0 g sugar, 1 g fiber, 5 g protein*

HAZELNUTS
Mildly sweet and very rich, this pick is the perfect partner for chocolate.

Per 1-oz serving *157 calories, 17 g fat (1 g saturated), 5 g carbs, 0 mg sodium, 0 g sugar, 3 g fiber, 4 g protein*

PINE NUTS
This tiny treasure supplies you with a hit of protein and a host of vitamins, like E and K, plus magnesium and iron.

Per 1-oz serving *178 calories, 17 g fat (TK g saturated), 5 g carbs, 0 mg sodium, 0 g sugar, 3 g fiber, 3 g protein*

PISTACHIOS
One ounce (about 49 pistachios) provides 13 percent of the standard recommended daily protein intake.

Per 1-oz serving *158 calories, 12.5 g fat (1.5 g saturated), 8 g carbs, 0 mg sodium, 0 g sugar, 3 g fiber, 6 g protein*

WALNUTS
They're also high in a plant-based omega-3 fat known as ALA, which can help fight chronic inflammation.

Per 1-oz serving *185 calories, 18.5 g fat (2 g saturated), 4 g carbs, 0 mg sodium, 0 g sugar, 2 g fiber, 4 g protein*

More Than Meats The Eye

No longer the dried-out meat you'd find only in a gas station, this snack staple is now made with higher quality sources.

How It's Made

Jerky is made by marinating thin strips of beef in a curing salt solution. The strips are hung on a stainless steel sheet, then cooked for 2.5 to 5 hours. All these steps give jerky a long shelf life, making it a perfect on-the-go high-protein snack.

Key Nutrition Info

Per the USDA, a typical 1-oz serving of plain beef jerky contains:

- ▶ 116 calories
- ▶ 7 g fat (3 g saturated fat)
- ▶ 3 g carbohydrates
- ▶ 9 g protein
- ▶ 0 g fiber
- ▶ 2.5 g sugar
- ▶ 506 mg sodium

Watch Out For

Because it's cured, the sodium content is super high. Just one ounce of standard jerky contains around 506 milligrams, according to the USDA—or 22 percent of the FDA's recommended daily amount. Another concern is nitrates—often added to jerkies as a preservative to prevent harmful bacteria from forming—which have been linked to cancer. And while jerky itself is low carb, added flavorings can amp up the carb and sugar content.

Healthy Jerky Checklist

When selecting jerky for a high-protein snack, make sure it fits this bill:

- ▶ Less than 400 mg sodium per serving
- ▶ Grass fed/organic
- ▶ Low sugar (no more than 8g per serving)
- ▶ All natural, whole-food-based ingredients
- ▶ Nitrate free and MSG free
- ▶ Opt for a credit-card-size, 1-oz serving
- ▶ Look for other jerky options beyond beef, including chicken, turkey, pork, salmon, and vegan varieties

The Bottom Line

Any jerky, whether it's meat or vegan, should be consumed in moderation and used as a snack when you don't have access to fresh fruit, vegetables, or other less shelf-stable items. Be diligent about your serving size or choose single-serving bags or bars to make it easy. And pair your snack with a side of hydration to help counteract the sodium content.

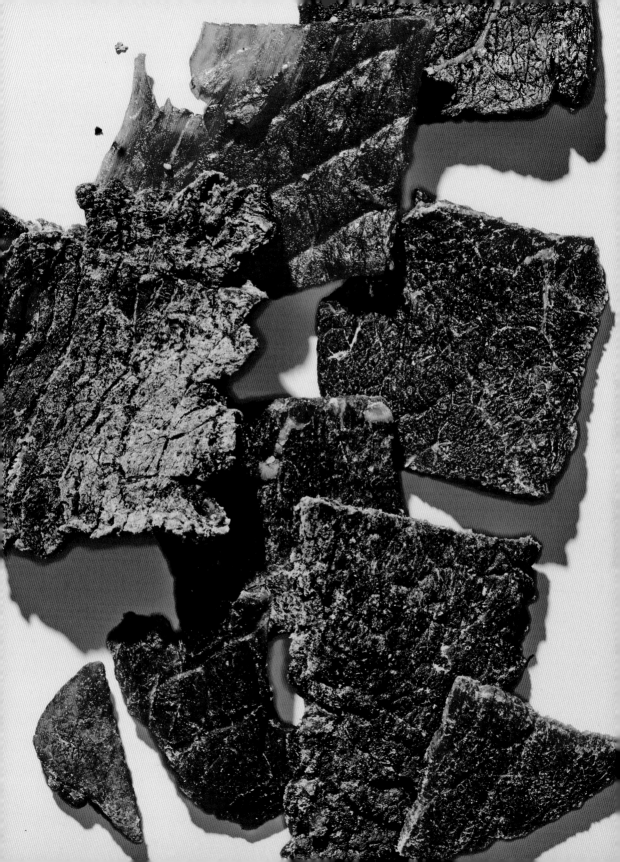

Index

WOMEN'S HEALTH

EDITOR-IN-CHIEF **Liz Baker Plosser**

EXECUTIVE EDITOR **Abigail Cuffey**

DESIGN DIRECTOR **Betsy Halsey**

MANAGING EDITOR **Laura McLaughlin**

DEPUTY VISUAL DIRECTOR **Dangi McCoy**

CHIEF FOOD DIRECTOR **Kate Merker**

DEPUTY FOOD EDITOR **Trish Clasen Marsanico**

ASSISTANT EDITOR **Samantha MacAvoy**

HEARST HOME

VICE PRESIDENT, PUBLISHER, HEARST BOOKS **Jacqueline Deval**

DEPUTY DIRECTOR, HEARST BOOKS **Nicole Fisher**

ART DIRECTOR **Laurene Chavez**

SENIOR PHOTO EDITOR **Cinzia Reale-Castello**

DEPUTY MANAGING EDITOR, HEARST BOOKS **Maria Ramroop**

SENIOR SALES & MARKETING COORDINATOR **Nicole Plonski**

PROJECT EDITOR **Liz Krieger**

PROJECT ART DIRECTOR **Jaclyn Loney**

DIGITAL IMAGE SPECIALIST **Ruth Vazquez**

COPY EDITORS **Dave Block, Vanessa Weiman**

INDEXER **Jay Krieder**

PRODUCTION CONSULTANT **Bill Rose**

PREPRESS CONSULTANT **Ray Chokov**

PUBLISHED BY HEARST

PRESIDENT & CHIEF EXECUTIVE OFFICER **Steven R. Swartz**

CHAIRMAN **William R. Hearst III**

EXECUTIVE VICE CHAIRMAN **Frank A. Bennack, Jr.**

HEARST MAGAZINES, INC.

PRESIDENT **Debi Chirichella**

GENERAL MANAGER, HEARST ENTHUSIAST & WELLNESS GROUP **Brian Madden**

GLOBAL CHIEF REVENUE OFFICER **Lisa Ryan Howard**

EDITORIAL DIRECTOR **Lucy Kaylin**

CHIEF FINANCIAL AND STRATEGY OFFICER **Regina Buckley**

CONSUMER GROWTH OFFICER **Lindsey Horrigan**

CHIEF PRODUCT & TECHNOLOGY OFFICER **Daniel Bernard**

PRESIDENT, HEARST MAGAZINES INTERNATIONAL **Jonathan Wright**

SECRETARY **Catherine A. Bostron**

PUBLISHING CONSULTANTS **Gilbert C. Maurer, Mark F. Miller**

This book is intended as a reference volume only, not as a medical manual. The information given here is designed to help you make informed decisions about your health. It is not intended as a substitute for any treatment that may have been prescribed by your doctor. If you suspect that you have a medical problem, we urge you to seek competent medical help.

Library of Congress Cataloging-in-Publication Data Available on Request

10 9 8 7 6 5 4 3 2 1

Published by Hearst Home, an imprint of
Hearst Books/Hearst Magazine Media, Inc.
300 W 57th Street
New York, NY 10019

Women's Health is a registered trademark of Hearst Magazines, Inc. Hearst Home, the Hearst Home logo, and Hearst Books are registered trademarks of Hearst Communications, Inc.

For information about custom editions, special sales, premium and corporate purchases: **hearst.com/magazines/hearst-books**

Printed in China
978-1-958395-61-5

JOIN WOMEN'S HEALTH+

Level up your health and fitness with exclusive fitness challenges and nutrition guides, 450+ streaming workouts, healthy recipes, unlimited website access, and so much more.

Sign up now at **womenshealthmag.com/joinpremium**

CREDITS

COVER Linda Xiao. Food styling: Rebecca Jurkevich. Prop styling: Maeve Sheridan. **Linda Xiao** (1, 6–7, 34–35, 55, 78, 111, 118) Food styling: Rebecca Jurkevich. Prop styling: Maeve Sheridan (112, 126, 138). **Chelsea Kyle** (2, 8, 31, 32, 50, 76, 87, 100, 104, 123, 166–167, back cover) Food styling: Tyna Hoang. Prop styling: Maeve Sheridan (59). **Joe Lingeman** (4, 48) Food styling: Rebecca Jurkevich (19, 38, 52, 64, 97), Food styling: Maggie Ruggiero (20–21, 24, 28, 36, 107, 148, 162–165, back cover). **Justin Steele/ Studio D** (5). **Nadine Greeff/Stocksy** (11, 16). **Nico Schinco** (12, 102) Food styling: Rebecca Jurkevich. Prop styling: Maeve Sheridan (12), Food styling: Hadas Smirnoff (99, 109, 142). **Getty Images** (15, 22, 70). **Mike Garten** (26, 152, 154, 157, 161) Food Styling: Simon Andrews. Prop Styling: Lis Engelhart (57, 80, 90), Food Styling: Christine Albano Prop Styling: Paige Hicks (75) Food Styling: Simon Andrews. Prop Styling: Christina Lane (95), Food Styling: Rebecca Jurkevich. Prop Styling: Lis Engelhart (125, 128). **Sam Kaplan** (40). **Ted&Chelsea** (43, 67). **Julia Gartland.** Food styling: Olivia Mack McCool (45, 140) Food styling: Lauren LaPenna. Prop styling: Summer Moore (83, 137), Food styling: Rebecca Jurkevich; Prop styling: Maeve Sheridan (85, 92, 121). Laura Murray. Food styling: Rebecca Jurkevich. Prop styling: Carla Gonzalez-Hart (47, 60, 62, 69, 133, 135, 150). **Alex Lau.** Food styling: Maggie Ruggiero (59, 88, 130), Food styling: Olivia Mack McCool (147). **Rocky Luten.** Food styling: Rebecca Jurkevich (72, 114). **Paola + Murrary** (116). **Ficca + Luciano** (144). **Danielle Daly** (159, back cover). **Victor Prado** (169)